Action in Perception

Representation and Mind
Hilary Putnam and Ned Block, editors

Action in Perception

Alva Noë

The MIT Press
Cambridge, Massachusetts
London, England

MIT Press books may be purchased at special quantitiy discounts for business or sales
promotional use. For information, please email special_sales@mitpress.mit.edu or
write to Special Sales Department, The MIT Press, 5 Cambridge Center, Cambridge, MA
02142.

This book was set in Stone and Stone sans by Kolam Information Services Pvt. Ltd,
Pondicherry, and printed and bound in the United States of America.

Library of Congress Cataloging-in-Publication Data

Noë, Alva.
    Action in perception / Alva Noë.
        p. cm. — (Representation and mind)
    Includes bibliographical references and index.
    ISBN 0-262-14088-8 (alk. paper)
    1. Perception (Philosophy) 2. Act (Philosophy) I. Title. II. Series.

B828.45.N64 2005   2004056464
121'.34—dc22

10   9   8   7   6   5   4   3   2

Contents

Preface

This is a book about perception and consciousness. It is written for philosophers and for cognitive scientists, but also for artists, and anyone else who is interested in the way we manage to make—or fail to make—sensory contact with the world around us. In it I argue that perception and perceptual consciousness depend on capacities for action and capacities for thought; perception is, I argue, a kind of thoughtful activity.

Philosophy flourishes in the midst of scientific research, not only because philosopical problems are in good measure empirical, but because scientific problems are in good measure philosophical. This book is intended to contribute to the interdisciplinary *natural philosophy* of mind.

Action in Perception has been written against the background of ongoing collaborations (and friendships) with Evan Thompson, Kevin O'Regan, and Susan Hurley. I would not have written this book if not for these collaborations; I acknowledge my debt to them here.

I first got interested in perception as a B.Phil. student in Oxford in the late eighties. My interest was stimulated by the work of three philosophers whose work I read and with whom I had contact in Oxford: Peter Strawson, John Hyman, and Peter Hacker. The title of this book refers to Strawson's paper "Causation in Perception."

I began my own research on perception a few years later, as a graduate student at Harvard. Although this book bears only a distant relation to the dissertation I wrote there under Hilary Putnam, this preface is an appropriate place for me to express my gratitude to him: his insightful criticism, and his energetic example, continue to guide my own work.

I also owe a debt of gratitude to Daniel Dennett, who directs the Center for Cognitive Studies at Tufts, where I spent a postdoctoral year in 1995–1996. Some preoccupations of this book—for example, Gibson's 'ecological' approach to perception—were topics of our conversations. Dennett repeatedly challenged me to make explicit the significance of these matters for cognitive science. I try to meet his challenge in this book.

Many other people have helped me write this book, either directly, or indirectly.

For critical discussion (or correspondence) that has shaped my thinking, I would like to thank Adrian Cussins, Hubert Dreyfus, Sean Kelly, Philip Pettit, and the late Francisco Varela.

For helpful criticism of earlier versions of material in this book, or for critical exchange on related matters, I would like to thank Jonathan Cole, Edward Harcourt, Matthew Henken, Pierre Jacob, Tori McGeer, Dominic Murphy, Erik Myin, Judith Baldwin Noë, Luiz Pessoa, Jean Michel Roy, Kyle Sanford, Eric Schwitzgebel, John Searle, and Stephen White. Bence Nanay provided useful detailed criticism of the whole book, for which I am grateful. Thanks also to the members of my fall 2003 UC Berkeley seminar on consciousness and life.

I owe a special debt to several former teachers and colleagues: Stanley Cavell, David Chalmers, the late Burton Dreben, Warren Goldfarb, David Hoy, Hidé Ishiguro, Robert May, and Charles Parsons. As a philosopher and writer, I engage in imagined dialogue with them on a regular basis.

This book was written with financial support from a University of California President's Fellowship in the Humanities, with the help of a Charles A. Ryskamp/ACLS Research Fellowship, and also with the support of faculty research funds of the University of California.

I am grateful to the members of the Institut Jean Nicod in Paris for welcoming me among them and providing a stimulating environment in which to work on this book during the fall and winter of 2002–2003.

I cannot imagine having written this book without Miriam Dym.

I dedicate this book to my father, Hans Noë.

A.N.
Berkeley
May 2004

Acknowledgments

I thank the copyright holders of the following papers for permission to reproduce selections in this book:

Thought and experience. *American Philosophical Quarterly* 36, no. 3 (July 1999): 257–265.

Is perspectival self-consciousness nonconceptual? *The Philosophical Quarterly* 52, no. 207 (April 2002): 185–194.

On what we see. *Pacific Philosophical Quarterly* 83, no. 1 (2002): 57–80.

Is the visual world a grand illusion? *Journal of Consciousness Studies* 9, no. 5/6: 1–12.

Perception and causation: The puzzle unraveled. *Analysis* 63, no. 2 (April 2003): 93–100.

Experience without the head. Forthcoming in *Perceptual Experience,* ed. T. S. Gendler and J. Hawthorne. Oxford: Oxford University, 2005.

I thank Daniel Simons and the publishers of the journal *Perception* for permission to reproduce figure 2.6. This image was originally published in:

Simons, D. J., and C. F. Chabris. 1999. Gorillas in our midst: Sustained inattentional blindness for dynamic events. *Perception* 28: 1059–1074.

It is really vain to express the nature of something. We notice effects, and a complete account of these effects would perhaps comprise the nature of this thing. We attempt in vain to describe the character of a man; but a description of his actions and his deeds will create for us a picture of his character.

—Goethe, *The Theory of Colours*

1 The Enactive Approach to Perception: An Introduction

The theory of the body is already a theory of perception.
—M. Merleau-Ponty

1.1 The Basic Idea

The main idea of this book is that perceiving is a way of acting. Perception is not something that happens to us, or in us. It is something we do. Think of a blind person tap-tapping his or her way around a cluttered space, perceiving that space by touch, not all at once, but through time, by skillful probing and movement. This is, or at least ought to be, our paradigm of what perceiving is. The world makes itself available to the perceiver through physical movement and interaction. In this book I argue that all perception is touch-like in this way: Perceptual experience acquires content thanks to our possession of bodily skills. *What we perceive* is determined by *what we do* (or what we know how to do); it is determined by what we are *ready* to do. In ways I try to make precise, we *enact* our perceptual experience; we act it out.

To be a perceiver is to understand, implicitly, the effects of movement on sensory stimulation. Examples are ready to hand. An object looms larger in the visual field as we approach it, and its profile deforms as we move about it. A sound grows louder as we move nearer to its source. Movements of the hand over the surface of an object give rise to shifting sensations. As perceivers we are masters of this sort of pattern of sensorimotor dependence. This mastery shows itself in the thoughtless automaticity with which we move our eyes, head and body in taking in what is around us. We spontaneously crane our necks, peer, squint, reach for our glasses, or draw near to get a better look (or better to handle, sniff, lick or listen to what interests us). The central claim of what I call *the enactive approach* is that our ability to perceive not only depends on, but is constituted by, our possession of this sort of sensorimotor knowledge.[1]

One implication of the enactive approach is that only a creature with certain kinds of bodily skills—for example, a basic familiarity with the sensory effects of eye or hand movements, and so forth—could be a perceiver.[2] This is because, in effect, perceiving is a kind of skillful bodily activity. It may also be that only a creature capable of at least some primitive forms of perception could be capable of self-movement. Specifically, self-movement depends on perceptual modes of self-awareness, for example, proprioception and also 'perspectival self-consciousness' (i.e., the ability to keep track of one's relation to the world around one).[3]

A second implication of the enactive approach is that we ought to reject the idea—widespread in both philosophy and science—that perception is a process *in the brain* whereby the perceptual system constructs an *internal representation* of the world. No doubt perception depends on what takes place in the brain, and very likely there are internal representations in the brain (e.g., content-bearing internal states). What perception is, however, is not a process in the brain, but a kind of skillful activity on the part of the animal as a whole. The enactive view challenges neuroscience to devise new ways of understanding the neural basis of perception and consciousness.[4] I return to this controversial topic in chapter 7.

This idea of perception as a species of skillful bodily activity is deeply counterintuitive. It goes against many of our preconceptions about the nature of perception. We tend, when thinking about perception, to make vision, not touch, our paradigm, and we tend to think of vision on a photographic model. You open your eyes and you are given, at once, a sharply focused impression of the present world in all its detail. On this view, the relation between moving and perceiving is only instrumental. It is like the relation between the lugging around of a camera and the resulting picture. The lugging is preliminary to and disconnected from the photograph itself. And so with perceiving. By moving yourself, you can come to occupy a vantage point from which, say, better to see your goal. And then, having seen your goal, you can better decide what to do. But the seeing, and the moving, have no more to do with each other than the photograph and the schlepping of the camera, or the boxer's left hook, and the training that preceded it. Which is to say, they have a lot to do with each other, but the relation is nonconstitutive: The effectiveness of the punch is strictly independent of how the boxer learned to do it, and the qualities of the picture are independent of how the camera ended up where it was.

Susan Hurley (1998) has aptly called this simple view of the relation between perception and action the input-output picture: Perception is input from world to mind, action is output from mind to world, thought is the mediating process. If the input-output picture is right, then it must be possible, at least in principle, to disassociate capacities for perception, action, and thought. The main claim of this book is that such a divorce is not possible. I doubt that it is even truly conceivable. All perception, I argue, is intrinsically active. Perceptual experience acquires content thanks to the perceiver's skillful activity. I also argue—but I don't turn to this until late in the book (chapter 6)—that all perception is intrinsically thoughtful. Blind creatures may be capable of thought, but thoughtless creatures could never be capable of sight, or of any genuine content-bearing perceptual experience.[5] Perception and perceptual consciousness are types of thoughtful, knowledgeable activity.

My aim in this initial chapter is to set out the book's central themes.

1.2   A Puzzle about Perception: Experiential Blindness

For those who see, it is difficult to resist the idea that being blind is like being in the dark. When we think of blindness this way, we imagine it as a state of blackness, absence and deprivation. We suppose that there is a gigantic hole in the consciousness of a blind person, a permanent feeling of incompleteness. Where there could be light, there is no light.

This is a false picture of the nature of blindness. The longterm blind do not experience blindness as a disruption or an absence. This is not because, as legend has it, smell, touch and hearing get stronger to compensate for the failure to see (although this may be true to some degree; see Kaufman, Théoret, and Pascual-Leone 2002). It's because there is a way in which the blind do not experience their blindness at all. Consider, you are unable visually to discern what takes place in the room next door, but you do not experience this inability as a gaping hole in your visual awareness. Likewise, you don't encounter the absence of the sort of olfactory information that would be present to a bloodhound as something missing in your sense of smell. Nor do you notice the absence of information about the part of the visual field that falls on the "blind spot" of your retina. In this same way the blind do not encounter their blindness as an absence.

It is easy to demonstrate that there are or could be forms of blindness that were not at all like being in the dark. Imagine that you are out in a fog so dense that no matter where you turn or how you strain you only experience a homogeneous whiteness. This is what psychologists call a *Ganzfeld* (Metzger 1930, described in Gibson 1979, 150–151). You can reproduce the experience of a Ganzfeld by placing half a Ping-Pong ball over each eye (Hochberg, Triebel, and Seaman 1951; Gibson and Wadell 1952; Block 2001). Gibson used this method to argue that stimulation of the retina by light is not sufficient for vision. For even though you enjoy a pattern of visual stimulation—in some sense, you see the Ganzfeld—you are in effect blind. You have visual impressions, but they are bleached of content.

The enactive view of perception predicts that there are, broadly speaking, two different kinds of blindness. First, there is blindness due to damage or disruption of the sensitive apparatus. This is the familiar sort of blindness. It would include blindness caused by cataracts, by retinal disease or injury, or by brain lesion in the visual cortex. Second, there is blindness due not to the absence of sensation or sensitivity, but rather to the person's (or animal's) inability to integrate sensory stimulation with patterns of movement and thought. Let's call this second kind of blindness *experiential blindness* because it is blindness despite the presence of something like normal visual sensation.

Does experiential blindness actually occur? If it does, then we must reject the input-output picture. To see is not just to have visual sensations, it is to have visual sensations that are integrated, in the right sort of way, with bodily skills. Experiential blindness would provide evidence for the enactive approach to perception.

There's good reason to believe that experiential blindness does occur. As an example, consider attempts to restore sight in congenitally blind individuals whose blindness is due to cataracts. Cataracts impair the eye's sensitivity by obstructing light on its passage to the retina. From the standpoint of the input-output picture, it would be natural to suppose that removing the cataract would be like sweeping aside the blinds, letting in the light and thus enabling normal vision. This is not in fact what the medical literature on this teaches us.[6] What we learn from the case studies is that the surgery restores visual *sensation*, at least to a significant degree, but that it does not restore sight. In the period immediately after the operation, patients suffer blindness despite rich visual sensations. That is to say, they suffer experiential blindness.

Consider a few examples. Gregory and Wallace describe a cataract-surgery patient, S.B.:

> S.B.'s first visual experience, when the bandages were removed, was of the surgeon's face. He described the experience as follows: He heard a voice coming from in front of him and to one side: he turned to the source of the sound and saw a "blur." He realized that this must be a face. Upon careful questioning, he seemed to think that he would not have known that this was a face if he had not previously heard the voice and known that voices came from faces. (1963, 366)

Sacks makes a similar observation of his patient Virgil:

> He seemed to be staring blankly, bewildered, without focusing, at the surgeon, who stood before him, still holding the bandages. Only when the surgeon spoke—saying "Well?"—did a look of recognition cross Virgil's face.
>
> Virgil told me later that in this first moment he had no idea what he was seeing. There was light, there was movement, there was color, all mixed up, all meaningless, a blur. Then out of the blur came a voice that said, "Well?" Then, and only then, he said, did he finally realize that this chaos of light and shadow was a face—and, indeed, the face of his surgeon. (1995, 114)

Finally, Valvo's patient made the following entry in his diary:

> after the operation, I saw the light of the doctor's probe, appearing like an atomic explosion on a background of black. Then I saw something which I understood afterwards was the doctor's hand and, clearly, his fingers; they seemed small and red (and to me it resembled the hand of the devil). . . . What I took to be black holes I recognized after about a month as windows in houses facing the hospital. (Valvo 1971, 9)

These patients suffer from experiential blindness, or so I propose. Their visual sensitivity is restored, to be sure. Each of them undergoes dramatic and robust visual impressions or sensations in the immediate aftermath of the surgery. But none of them, in having these sensations, has acquired the ability to see, at least not in anything like the normal sense. The visual impressions they now receive remain confusing and uninformative to them, like utterances in a foreign language. They have sensations, but the sensations don't add up to experiences with representational content.

The existence of experiential blindness is of great importance. It demonstrates that merely to be given visual impressions is not yet to be made to see. To see one must have visual impressions that one *understands*. This is brought out forcibly in connection with Gregory and Wallace's S.B. They write, concerning S.B.'s state about a month after his operation:

At first impression he seemed like a normally sighted person, though differences soon became obvious. When he sat down he would not look round or scan the room with his eyes; indeed he would generally pay no attention to visual objects unless his attention were called to them, when he would peer at whatever it was with extreme concentration. (Gregory and Wallace 1963, 364)

S.B. has visual impressions, but he lacks, at least in part, a practical understanding of their significance for movement and thought. The point is not only that S.B. lacks the ability to use his impressions to guide movement, although this is true. In normal perceivers, sensation is smoothly integrated with capacities for thought, and for movement; so, for example, we naturally turn our eyes to objects of interest, we modulate our sensations with movement in a way that is responsive to thought and situation. A sharp sound makes us turn in the direction from which the sound emanates. A ball rushes toward us and we reflexively duck. A person speaks to us, we turn to him or her. In this sort of way, and in countless ways like this, sensory impressions are immediately coupled with spontaneous movement. This coupling is missing for S.B. and the other patients. S.B.'s deficit, however, is more far-reaching even than this; S.B.'s inability to use what he sees to guide movements is caused by what is in effect an inability to see (experiential blindness). S.B. lacks understanding of the sensorimotor significance of his impressions; he lacks knowledge of the way the stimulation varies as he moves or would move. As a result, or so I propose, his impressions are without content and he is, to a substantial degree, blind.

Defenders of the input-output picture may be skeptical. Perhaps, they might argue, one can grant that the newly post-operative patients are blind, but without conceding that they are *experientially* blind. After all, there would seem to be evidence that their difficulty stems not so much from abnormal sensorimotor integration, as from abnormal *sensations*. Look at how they describe their experience. Sack's Virgil reports encountering movement, color, "all meaningless, a blur," and Valvo's patient describes impressions of atomic explosions on a background of dark. These aren't normal visual sensations. They are clearly abnormal. This line of objection may be strengthened by considering that inactivity of retina and visual cortex could lead to some degree of stunting of the development of neural connections needed for mature adult vision. Until these possibilities are eliminated, the skeptic can insist that we are not entitled to treat the condition of these patients as *experiential* blindness (i.e., as blindness due to lack of sensorimotor knowledge rather than to lack of perceptual sensitivity). To establish genuine experiential blindness, we need to control for changes in the quality of visual impressions themselves. Until we can do this, we have no argument for the enactive approach and no argument against the input-output picture.

This objection has some force. In section 1.3 I turn to an example of putative experiential blindness that is not vulnerable to this criticism. Taken together the two examples make a strong case for experiential blindness, and so for the enactive approach.

1.3 Being Blinded by What You See

Glasses, or spectacles, belong to the humdrum everyday technology of perception. One of the most common kinds of glasses, or corrective lenses, are for myopia (or nearsightedness). In myopia, light from distant objects, which enters the eye in parallel rays, is brought to a focus before the retina, rather than on it. Light from nearer objects does not consist in parallel rays and is brought to a focus on the retina. What glasses for myopia do is bend light from distant objects so that it enters the eye at the same angle as light from nearer objects, thus allowing it to be brought to a focus on the retina.

What happens if glasses consist of prisms that distort or bias the light entering the eyes in strange or unnatural ways? Suppose you construct lenses so that light from objects on the left enters the eye just as light coming from an object on the right would enter the eye if you were not wearing the lenses. A left-side object would thus stimulate right-side retina, and also right-side brain (that is to say, the parts of the retina and brain normally stimulated by objects on the right). It is reasonable to suppose that in a case such as this you would have an experience as of an object on the right side.

In fact, as experiments by Stratton (1897), Kohler ([1951] 1964), and later Taylor (1962) demonstrate, this is not what happens, or at least not what happens right away. The initial effect of inverting glasses of this sort is not an inversion of the content of experience (an inversion of what is seen) but rather a partial disruption of seeing itself. Inverting lenses give rise to experiential blindness. Consider what one subject, K, wrote of his initial experiences in Kohler's experiment with displacing spherical prism spectacles:

During visual fixations, every movement of my head gives rise to the most unexpected and peculiar transformations of objects in the visual field. The most familiar forms seem to dissolve and reintegrate in ways never before seen. At times, parts of figures run together, the spaces between disappearing from view: at other times, they run apart, as if intent on deceiving the observer. Countless times I was fooled by these extreme distortions and taken by surprise when a wall, for instance, suddenly appeared to slant down to the road, when a truck I was following with my eyes started to bend, when the road began to arch like a wave, when houses and trees seemed to topple down, and so forth. I felt as if I were living in a topsy-turvy world of houses crashing down on you, of heaving roads, and of jellylike people. (Kohler [1951] 1964)

K is not completely blind, to be sure; he recognizes the trucks, the trees, and so forth. But nor is he completely able to see. His visual world is distorted, made unpredictable and topsy-turvy. To this extent, K suffers blindness. Crucially, the kind of blindness K suffers is not caused by any defect in sensation. K receives normal stimulation. The light reaching his eyes is sharply focused and fully information-bearing. He receives exactly the stimulation he would receive were he looking at an object in a different spatial location without the inverting lenses. The inability to see normally stems not from the character of the stimulation, but rather from the perceiver's understanding (or rather failure of understanding) of the stimulation.

This is exactly what the enactive approach would lead us to expect, as O'Regan and I have argued (O'Regan and Noë 2001a,b; Noë 2002a; see also Hurley and Noë 2003a). The basis of perception, on our enactive, sensorimotor approach, is implicit practical knowledge of the ways movement gives rise to changes in stimulation. When you put on the distorting lenses, the patterns of dependence between movement and stimulation are altered. This alteration has the effect of abrogating sensorimotor knowledge or skill, even though there is no change in the intrinsic character of stimulation. As a consequence, movements of the eye and head give rise to surprising and unanticipated changes in sensory stimulation. The result is not *seeing differently*, but failing to see.

Strictly speaking, the goggles do not produce *total* experiential blindness. This is because the only sensorimotor dependencies that are affected are those pertaining to aspects of spatial content. For example, left-right reversing prisms do not affect one's sense of up and down (although they do affect one's sense, say, of the speed with which the visual world "swings by" as one moves one's eyes). Moreover, left-right reversing goggles do not affect one's sense of light and dark, color, and so on. When you put on left-right reversing goggles, you enjoy *some* perceptual experience. For example, you can tell whether the lights are on. This is not surprising, given that the goggles don't change *all* the patterns of sensorimotor dependence, only those that are related to spatial orientation.

The enactive view would also lead us to expect that vision will be restored once one comes to grips with the new patterns of sensorimotor dependence. The experimental literature supports this. Kohler's reports suggest that adaptation occurs in stages. The first stage of adaptation is the experience of inverted content. Now objects on the left do indeed look just as if they are on the right. Your visual experience has acquired nonveridical content. But this state of partial adaptation is highly unstable. Your left hand may look as if it is on the right, but it continues to *feel* as if it is on the left (Hurley and Noë 2003a). And when you snap your fingers, the sound of your "hand on the right" seems to come from the left. At the next stage of adaptation, visual experience "captures" auditory and proprioceptive experience, resolving conflicts between these sensory modalities in favor of vision. The object on the left not only looks as if it is on the right, but it now sounds and feels as if it is too. If subjects are allowed (indeed required) to actively engage with and explore their environment, a third stage of adaptation comes about in which experience comes to "right itself" and veridicality is restored. Now objects on the left look as though they are on the left, even though they continue, as before, to activate retinal and brain areas associated with right-placed stimuli. This is the final stage of adaptation. (For discussion, see Hurley and Noë 2003a.)

From the standpoint of the enactive view, this is an extraordinarily important phenomenon, a powerful illustration of the fact that perceptual experience acquires content as a result of sensorimotor knowledge. I return to some of these issues in chapter 3. For now the point is this: Once full adaptation has been achieved, the result of *removing* the lenses is comparable to the initial effects of putting them on. Taking the glasses off induces exactly the same kind of experiential blindness, and for exactly the same reasons that putting them on did at first: The glasses (or their absence) cause a sudden abrogation of the patterns of dependence of sensation and movement. Kohler's subject describes the effects of taking the lenses off as follows:

As I begin to move and walk about, the room begins to move too. What I am experiencing are the apparent movements of the objects around me. As I approach one of them, it seems to move to the right. I reach out for it and touch—air: my arm has completely missed it, passed to the left of it. . . . Even more peculiar are the relative changes inside the room. When I move my head (vertically or horizontally), not a single point remains stationary in relation to another point. If a certain point moves along with me in the visual field, then some other point will infallibly move in the opposite direction, as if indicating to me in no uncertain terms that it is not the least bit bound by what the other points appear to be doing at the time.

The world I am in seems to have become a total chaos of continuously changing distances, directions, movements, and Gestalten. Nothing remains stable and the experience is so confusing that I am unable to detect what laws the transformations abide by . . . everything remains without rhyme or reason. There is no such thing as *a* size or *a* movement; as soon as I move my body or my head, any object is apt to become smaller or larger, stationary or mobile. (Kohler [1951] 1964, 65)

The effect of removing the lenses, then, is to produce nonveridical, distorted, chaotic visual impressions, even though the patterns of visual sensation now produced are exactly as they were before the lenses were first put on. Objects on the left stimulate the parts of the eye and brain that have always supported the sensory experience of leftness. The inability normally to perceive is the result not of changes in the intrinsic character or location of the sensory stimulation, but rather of the induced breakdown in our mastery or control over the ways sensory stimulation changes as a function of movement.

To summarize, experiential blindness exists and is important for two reasons. First, it lends support for the enactive view. Genuine perceptual experience depends not only on the character and quality of stimulation, but on our exercise of sensorimotor knowledge. The disruption of this knowledge does not leave us with experiences we are unable to put to use. It leaves us without experience. For mere sensory stimulation to constitute perceptual experience—that is, for it to have genuine world-presenting content—the perceiver must possess and make use of *sensorimotor knowledge*.

Second, it provides a counter example to the more traditional input-output picture. Kant ([1781–1787] 1929) famously said that intuitions without concepts are blind. The present point is that intuitions—patterns of stimulation—without knowledge of the sensorimotor significance of those intuitions, are blind. Crucially, the knowledge in question is practical knowledge; it is know-how.[7] To perceive you must be in possession of *sensorimotor bodily skill*.

1.4 The Joys of Seeing

A natural line of objection to the enactive approach goes like this: True, our perceptual capacities are bound up with bodily skill and action. We use our eyes to guide our movements and to enable action. But that is not always the case. Sometimes we see not in order to act, but just in order to know, or to enjoy our experiences of seeing. When you lie back and watch the passing clouds, or when you visit an art gallery, or watch TV, you are not using visual skills for purposes of action. Pylyshyn (2001) has made this point; he adds that "much of what we see guides our action only indirectly by changing what we believe and perhaps what we want" (999).

This criticism of the enactive view would seem to gain support from the study of neurological disorders of vision. Patients with *optic ataxia* (resulting from lesions in posterior parietal cortex) are unable to make use of what they see to guide movements. As Milner and Goodale write, "Yet despite the failure of these patients to orient their hands, to scale their grip appropriately, or to reach towards the right location, they have comparatively little difficulty in giving perceptual reports of the orientation and location of the very objects they fail to grasp" ([1998] 2002, 520). Milner and Goodale argue that there are two largely autonomous visual systems. Damage to the dorsal stream (from striate to posterior parietal cortex) impairs visuomotor skill without harming vision or visual awareness as such. Damage to the ventral stream (from striate to inferotemporal cortex), in contrast, can produce striking visual agnosias, impairing object recognition and judgments of size, orientation and location, while leaving visuomotor skill largely intact. Their subject D.F., for example, showed excellent visually guided control of grasp, reaching, and hand posture in general. According to Milner and Goodale, "Yet when she was asked to use her finger and thumb to make a perceptual judgment of the object's width on a separate series of trials, D.F.'s responses were unrelated to the actual stimulus dimensions, and showed high variation from trial to trial" ([1998] 2002, 520–522). This neurological evidence suggests that although some facets of vision are bound up with visuomotor skill, this is not true of vision as a whole. The enactive approach, it would seem, exaggerates the importance of action in perception.

This criticism rests on a misunderstanding of the enactive approach. The basic claim of the enactive approach is that the perceiver's ability to perceive is constituted (in part) by sensorimotor knowledge (i.e., by practical grasp of the way sensory stimulation varies as the perceiver moves). The enactive approach does not claim that perception is *for* acting or for guiding action. The existence of optic ataxia, therefore, does not undercut the enactive view, for from the fact that a patient suffers optic ataxia, it doesn't follow they he or she lacks the relevant sensorimotor knowledge. What would undercut the enactive approach would be the existence of perception in the absence of the bodily skills and sensorimotor knowledge which, on the enactive view, are constitutive of the ability to perceive. Could there be an entirely inactive, an *inert* perceiver?

Before we turn to this question, consider a simpler worry. Paralysis is certainly not a form of blindness. But isn't that precisely what the enactive view requires, that the paralyzed be experientially blind? No. The enactive view requires that perceivers possess a range of pertinent sensorimotor skills. It seems clear that quadriplegics have the pertinent skills. Quadriplegics can move their eyes and head, and to some extent, at least with help from technology, they can move their bodies with respect to the environment (e.g., by using a wheelchair). More important, paralysis does not undermine the paralyzed person's practical understanding of the ways movement and sensory stimulation depend on each other. Even the paralyzed, whose range of movement is restricted, understand, implicitly and practically, the significance of movement for stimulation. They understand, no less than those who are not disabled, that movement of the eyes to the left produces rightward movement across the visual field, and so forth. Paralyzed people can't do as much as people who are not paralyzed, but they can do a great deal; whatever the scope of their limitations, they draw on a wealth of sensorimotor skill that informs and enables them to perceive.

Quadriplegics, who are without sensation as well as movement, live extremely active lives. As the clinical neurophysiologist Jonathan Cole remarks, "Try balancing in a chair without any sensation from the neck down" (personal communication, but see Cole 2004). Quadriplegics are continuously engaged in the task of orienting themselves in relation to the world around them and to gravity (as Cole 2004 discusses).[8]

There is in fact strong empirical evidence that a more thoroughgoing paralysis—for example, of the eyes themselves—would cause blindness. In normal perceivers, the eyes are in nearly constant motion, engaging in saccades (sharp, ballistic movements) and microsaccades several times a second. If the eyes were to cease moving, they'd lose their receptive power. In particular, it has been shown that images stabilized on the retina fade from view (Ditchburn and Ginsborg 1952; Riggs et al. 1953; Krauskopf 1963; Yarbus 1967). This is probably an instance of the more general phenomenon of *sensory fatigue* thanks to which we do not continuously feel our clothing on our skin, the glasses resting on the bridge of our nose, or a ring on our finger. This suggests that some minimal amount of eye and body movement is necessary for perceptual sensation.

There is also developmental evidence that normal vision depends not only on movement of the body relative to the environment, but on *self-actuated* movement. Held and Hein (1963) performed an experiment in which two kittens were harnessed to a carousel. One of the kittens was harnessed in such a way that it stood firmly on the ground. The other kitten was suspended in the air. As the one kitten walked, both kittens moved in a circle. As a result, they received identical visual stimulation, but only one of them received that stimulation as a result of self-movement. Remarkably (but not surprisingly from an enactive viewpoint), only the self-moving kitten developed normal depth perception (not to mention normal paw-eye coordination). From an enactive standpoint, we can venture an explanation for this: Only through *self*-movement can one *test* and so *learn* the relevant patterns of sensorimotor dependence.[9]

There are, however, deeper and more compelling reasons to be skeptical of the very idea that there could be a truly passive, inert perceiver. One of the main aims of this book is to demonstrate this. A few preliminary remarks now can set us on the path.

The extraordinary case of Ian Waterman, documented by Jonathan Cole (1991), serves as an illustration. Waterman, as a young man, took ill with a virus that produced a dramatic and far-reaching neuropathy. Although his motor nerves remained unaffected, he lost all sensation from the neck down, except for the sensation of pain (e.g., pin pricks) and temperature. In particular, he lost what is sometimes called "the sixth sense," namely, the sense of movement and position known as proprioception and kinaesthesis. Waterman was initially, in effect, paralyzed. Despite the fact that he possessed a normally functioning motor system, he was unable to bring his limbs and body under his control. In the absence of proprioceptive feedback, he was unable to move. Eventually, he regained a good measure of motor skill by learning to substitute vision for muscular sense. By intense visual concentration, he was able to control his body movements. However, if he were put into a position in which he could not view his body (say, reclining on a couch), or if the lights were to go out, he would collapse to the ground, unable to move. As Cole says, in the case of Ian Waterman, for his body to be out of sight was, literally, for it to be out of mind.

What would Ian Waterman have done if he had been blind as well? Let's consider a made-up case. Suppose that you suffer from a neuropathy like Waterman's—that is to say, that you have lost all sense of movement, position and posture—but imagine that you are, in addition, deaf and blind. Let's further imagine that you have *normal* sensation from the neck down. Strictly speaking, this last detail is not consistent with the supposition that you lack all proprioception, since proprioception depends in part on cutaneous sensitivity (in addition to the activation of muscle spindles and tendon receptors). But let's put this complication aside and imagine that you have normal tactile sensation, but that you lack a sense of movement, position, and posture, and that you are deaf and blind. To imagine this, then, is to imagine that you are inert, that you are radically unable to act with your body. It is to imagine that your body has been lost to you as an animated part of yourself.

Now let us ask, would you be able to perceive by touch? Could you enjoy tactile experience of the world around you? By hypothesis your cutaneous sensory receptors are intact, so there is no question whether you can feel, that is, have tactile sensations. The question is, in having tactile sensations, would you perceive how things are around you?

In general, there are reasons to doubt that tactile sensation or feeling is sufficient for tactile perception. To perceive by touch, for example, the rectangularity of something you hold in your hands, or the layout of furniture in a room (as a blind person might, by moving around and reaching and touching) is not merely to have certain feelings or sensations. After all,

the rectangularity is not captured by specific sensations. The
tary sensation or feel of a rectangle. The rectangularity is made
you, in touch, by your active touching (probing, prodding, st
bing, squeezing) with your hands. What informs you of the sh... ... what
you feel or hold is not the intrinsic character of your sensations, but rather
your implicit understanding of the organization or structure of your sensations. The shape is made available thanks to the way in which your
sensations co-vary or would co-vary with actual or possible movements. In
perceiving the thing as rectangular, you understand, implicitly, that, for
example, if you move your hands like *so*, you'll encounter corners that
stand in a certain relation to each other, and so forth. The same sort of
point can be made about the tactile perception of the layout of furniture
in the room. Your tactile impression that things are arranged thus and such
consists not in the sensations in your hands and feet, but in the way those
sensations result from attentive movement through the space. What is
informative is the fact that you bump your foot here, that you cannot press
forward there, and so on. You perceive the furniture layout when you
understand the way your sensations are fixed as a function of movement
through the space. In this way, sensation and sensorimotor knowledge
work together to produce the perception of the spatial layout of the room.

For this reason it seems plausible that feeling alone is not sufficient to
enable you to learn about or discover the properties of objects or layouts
around you. It is altogether unclear, in the extreme case of inert perception
I am imagining, that you would be able to learn how things are around
you, for you would be unable to probe in response to sensations, and so
would be unable, even in thought, to coordinate them. How could you
perceive the object *as rectangular* without moving it across your body
surfaces, or without moving your body surfaces across it?

One response is that you could at least perceive *heat*, say, or *texture*. For
these simple tactile qualities, it might seem that feeling is sufficient for tactile perception. This is plausible, but we need to be cautious. You will have
sensations, to be sure, but will they amount to perception of how things
are, even with respect to heat or texture? Because you are completely inert,
you may be unable to localize your sensations on your body. Suppose
someone presses, say, a warm spoon against your thigh. What will you
experience? A feeling of warmth on your thigh? Or merely a feeling of
warmth? In either case, your experience will be confined to the character

of your own sensations. Your would-be perception of the warmth of something will collapse into the mere sensation of warmth somewhere (perhaps conjoined with the inference that that sensation is likely to have an external source). Such a sensation-plus-guesswork falls short of constituting perceptual experience with content (at least of the normal sort). At best, it would seem, it is a primitive antecedent of the latter.

Remember, what is in question here is the experience of one who is radically inert. Ian Waterman, and others with similar conditions, are not radically inert. They *are* able to locate sensations of heat on, say, their legs; without proprioception (or vision), they are unable to locate the leg, however, in surrounding space. My suggestion is that for one whose sensations bear no familiar dependence on patterns of movement, even this localization on the surfaces of one's own body would be impossible.

One objection might be that sometimes mere touch is enough for perception. A sense of touch, for example, signals the presence of a fly, or some other object. Yes, and no. We *do* experience the presence and location of a fly, say, by the merest sense of touch on the skin, but this is only because we also possess the sensorimotor skills needed to interpret that touch as referring to a type of movement or position in space. We spontaneously withdraw our arm from the touch, for example, and in this way we give expression to the understanding that such a movement of the arm is a movement *away* from the point of contact with the fly. What would it be to experience the touch as an instant of contact with the fly, if one were not also able, thus, to understand the way movements would alter one's relation to that point in space?

The enactive view insists that mere feeling is not sufficient for perceptual experience (i.e., for experience with world-representing content).[10] O'Shaughnessy (2000) has argued that it is not even necessary for perceptual experience.[11] You could perceive the presence of a wall by reaching out and pressing it with your numb hand. Your ability to do that probably depends on your having feelings elsewhere. But, as O'Shaughnessy points out, those feelings are not part of your experience; they do not belong to the scope of your attention in perceiving the wall by touch. This point is nicely illustrated by the case of a blind person perceiving by means of a cane. There is no feeling at the end of the cane, yet it is with the end of the cane that the blind person makes contact with the world. It is probable that the ability thus to perceive depends on one's capacity for sensation (say, in the hand that holds the cane). But crucially, sensations in your hand are *not* constituents of your cane-based perceptual experience of the environment.

On the enactive view, all perception is in these respects like touch. Mere sensation, mere stimulation, falls short of perceptual awareness. As stated earlier, for perceptual sensation to constitute experience—that is, for it to have genuine representational content—the perceiver must possess and make use of *sensorimotor knowledge*. To imagine a truly inert perceiver is to imagine someone without the sensorimotor knowledge needed to enact perceptual content.

1.5 Action in Perception in Cognitive Science

The enactive approach to perception draws on a number of distinct traditions in philosophy, psychology, and cognitive science. The touch-like character of vision plays an important role in Merleau-Ponty's philosophical writing ([1948] 1973, [1945] 1962), and in the writing of other phenomenologists (e.g., Jonas 1966). Berkeley ([1709] 1975), Poincaré ([1902] 1952, [1905] 1958), Husserl ([1907] 1997), and Evans (1982) offer accounts of the spatial content of perceptual experience that anticipate elements of the enactive approach. (I turn to this topic in chapter 3.) In cognitive science, both the motor theory of perception (Berthoz [1997] 2000; Jeannerod 1997) and Gibson's ecological approach to perception (Gibson 1979) lay great emphasis on perception as an activity. Several other influential thinkers have emphasized and developed, in different ways, the sensorimotor basis of perception—for example, MacKay (1967, 1973); Arbib (1989); Koenderink (1984a,b); Varela (Varela, Thompson, and Rosch 1991; Maturana and Varela 1987); and O'Regan (1992). In addition, there has been a great deal of interest in recent cognitive science on the relation between perception and action—for example, Ballard (1991, 1996, 2002); Thompson (Thompson, Palacios, and Varela 1992; Thompson 1995); Humphrey (1992); Churchland, Ramachandran, and Sejnovksy (1994); Kelso (1995); Cotteril (1995, 2001); Clark (1997, 1999); Hurley (1998); Järvilehto (1998a,b, 1999, 2000); O'Regan and Noë (2001a,b,c); Noë (2002a,b).[12] A hallmark of this new work is the idea that the relation between perception and action is more complicated than traditional approaches have supposed.

In this section I give a brief sketch of some lines of thought that converge on the enactive approach. I don't try to give anything like a complete survey.[13] The enactive view gains indirect support from these disparate research lines. Importantly, care is required before the enactive approach is identified with any of these disparate strands. Most recent work on the relation of perception and action stops short of making the constitutive claim that defines the enactive standpoint: It does not treat perception as a kind of action or skillful activity (or as drawing on a kind of sensorimotor knowledge); rather it treats (a good deal of) perception as *for* the guidance of action.

One important source of the idea that perception and action are more tightly connected than the input-output picture tends to suppose is comparative and evolutionary work on perception. It seems probable that vision, for example, evolved as a mechanism of motor control. Certainly it is the case that in simple organisms the absorption of light may have the effect of modulating locomotion thanks to direct biochemical linkages (Bruce and Green [1985] 1990; Humphrey 1992). As an example, consider the phototactic water beetle (*Dytiscidae*). (This example is discussed in Milner and Goodale 1998, 6. See also Schone 1962.) The absorption of light directly produces a modulation of swimming behavior, leading the organism toward the light. In a normal aquatic environment this tends to lead it upward to the air it needs to survive. But the animal will swim to the bottom if that's where a light source is placed, resulting in death. A well-known example is the visual system of the frog, where certain patterns of stimulation are thought to activate "a fly detection response" leading to a darting out of the tongue in the direction of the stimulus (Lettvin et al. 1959). It is probable that our own sophisticated visual capacities develop from these humble sensorimotor beginnings.

A second important source is work in neurology, and psychology, on the existence of two functionally separable visual systems in the brain, one subserving vision and the other subserving the control of visually guided behavior. As mentioned earlier, the neurological evidence is striking: Visual agnosics may have normal visuomotor skills in the absence of normal perception and patients with optic ataxia can make normal perceptual judgments in the absence of normal visuomotor skill (Milner and Goodale 1995; but see Rossetti, Pisella, and Vighetta 2003). There is also psychological evidence that supports this two-systems approach. In particular, evidence exists that vision may guide motor behavior (say, pointing) unconsciously (or implicitly). Subjects may have no access to the visual information, in the sense that they are unable to *say* what they see, even though this information is exploited to guide movement. Bridgeman and his colleagues, for example, gave subjects the task of pointing at a target that was displaced and then extinguished (Bridgeman et al. 1979). They were asked whether the target had been displaced or not. Subjects tended to point correctly, whether or not they noticed a displacement. In a later study, they created an illusion that a target had jumped by moving a background frame in which the target was presented. Pointing accuracy was not affected by the illusion of displacement (Bridgeman, Kirch, and Sperling 1981). Apparent displacement of the target affected only perception, not pointing. In a second condition they allowed subjects to adjust the target's real (as opposed to induced) motion so that it moved in phase with the frame and came to look stationary. Despite this perceived lack of displacement, subjects successfully pointed to the real displacement. In this condition, real displacement went unperceived but affected the motor system. In this way, Bridgeman and his colleagues demonstrate that perceptual and motor functions are successfully dissociated. (For a review of this and other research on the two-systems hypothesis, see Bridgeman 1992 and Bridgeman et al. 2000.)

The significance, for the enactive approach, of this dissociation of perception and perceptual-guidance of action is delicate. The existence of a "how" (dorsal) stream, dedicated to the visual guidance of action, would seem to lend some measure of support to the enactive approach, insofar as it gives additional support to the claim that there are strong constitutive links between perception and action. However, the existence of a "what" (ventral) stream, dedicated to perceptual representation, experience, and identification, would seem to indicate that at least some aspects of perception are independent of links to motor systems.

In fact, Milner and Goodale's two visual systems hypothesis is, at best, orthogonal to the basic claims of the enactive approach. The enactive approach is not committed to the idea that vision is for the guidance of action, so neither the fact that some visual processing *is* for the guidance of action, nor the fact that some visual processing *is not*, has any direct bearing on the enactive approach. From the standpoint of the enactive approach, all perceptual representation, whether the result of dorsal or ventral stream activity, depends on the perceiver's deployment of sensorimotor skills.

One idea that serves to guide investigation into the active character of perception is the recognition that some of the most difficult challenges faced by traditional approaches to perception are, in a sense, debts incurred precisely by a failure to make room, in an account of perception, for the role of action.

As an example, note that traditional approaches to vision suppose that the problem of vision is one of "inverse optics," namely, to produce a description of the three-dimensional environmental layout from a projection of that environment in two dimensions on the retina (Marr 1982). The problem, as is well known, is ill posed. Just as a small object nearby can project the same image as a large object far away, so, in general, one cannot "read off" a description of the scene from the information made available in the retinal image. When the problem is framed this way, the brain's task is frequently supposed to be that of forming a hypothesis (e.g., an inference to the best explanation) as to the distal causes of proximal stimuli (e.g., Fodor 1975).

But why should we suppose that the data for vision is the content of the retinal image? If we think of the perceiver not as the brain-photoreceptor system, but rather as the whole animal, situated in the environment, free to move around and explore, then we can take seriously the possibility that the data for vision (as distinct from data for the photoreceptor) are not the content of a static snapshot-like retinal image. At the very least, the animal or brain has access to the "dynamic flow" of continuously varying retinal information. Optic flow contains information that is not available in single retinal images (Gibson 1979). For example, expanding optic field flow indicates that the observer is approaching a fixed point; contracting optic field flow indicates that he or she is moving away from a fixed point (Gibson 1979, 227).

This suggests that part of what has made the computational problem of vision such a difficult one is that it is framed in an artificially restrictive way. Perceivers aren't confined to their retinal images in the way traditional theorists have supposed.

Gibson took these points further. He argued that the animal has access not only to information contained in optic flow, but also to information about the way optic flow varies as a function of movement. When we move through a cluttered environment, for example, one object may come to occlude another. But occlusion, as Gibson noticed, is reversible (1979, chap. 5). By tracing movements back, you can bring an occluded surface back into view. In perceptual activity the perceiver is thus able to differentiate mere occlusion from obliteration. This is an example of the way it is possible for the animal to explore the structure of the flow of sensory changes and to discern in this structure *invariant* properties of the environment. Gibson also held that his 'ecological' approach can handle the problem of inverse optics mentioned earlier. This problem turns out to be a consequence of the optional assumption that the data for vision is confined to the retinal image. For an active animal, it is easy to disambiguate a large but distant object from a near but large one.

Gibson went further than this, however. He argued that just as there is a fit between an animal and the environmental niche it occupies, thanks to the coevolution of animal and niche, so there is a tight *perceptual attunement* between animal and environment. Because of this attunement, animals (as embodied wholes, not as brain systems attached to photoreceptors) are directly sensitive to the features of the world that afford the animal opportunities for action (what Gibson 1979, chap. 8, called "affordances"). For the active animal, the ground is directly perceived as walk-uponable, and the tree stump as sit-uponable. The theory of affordances is very controversial, as is Gibson's theory of direct perception more generally. He has been roundly criticized by, among others, Ullman (1980) and Fodor and Pylyshyn (1981). I do not endorse Gibson's views across the board. However, many of the criticisms leveled against him can be answered pretty easily. In fact, from the standpoint of the enactive approach, it is possible to reconstruct certain of his most controversial claims (e.g., the theory of affordances and his account of the so-called ambient optic array).

We return to these themes in chapters 3 and 4. For now the crux is this: There is a solidifying consensus in cognitive science that information available to an active animal greatly outstrips information available to a static retina, and that it is a mistake to suppose that the animal's data for visual perception are confined to the contents of the retinal image.

Once we adopt an active approach to perception, treating the active animal as the subject of perception, we are led to question the assumption (made by Marr and most theorists working in the computational school) that vision is a process whereby the brain produces an internal representation of the world (of what is seen). Churchland, Ramachandran, and Sejnowski (1994) call this the theory of pure vision, namely, the doctrine that vision is a matter of generating a detailed internal representation of the visual world on the basis of information available at the retina alone. If vision evolved for the purpose of enabling creatures to get by in a hostile environment (e.g., to facilitate the famous four Fs, etc.), then why assume, by building it into the definition, as it were, that vision requires the construction of a detailed internal representation? Presumably that is an empirical matter (Noë, Pessoa, and Thompson 2000).

An active approach to perception raises a more significant concern. If the animal is present *in* the world, with access to environmental detail by movements—that is, if it is active, embodied, environmentally situated—then why does it need to go to the trouble of producing internal representations good enough to enable it, so to speak, to act as if the world were not immediately present? Surely we sometimes need to think about the world in the world's absence (when it's dark, say, or when we're blind, or not at the location we're interested in), and for such purposes we must (in some sense) represent the world in thought. But what reason is there to think that this is the case in standard perceptual contexts? In many situations, we need only move our eyes, or move our head, or turn around, to get whatever information we need about the environment. How many bookshelves are there in your room? You don't need to have an internal representation to answer; you need only be able to turn around and take a look. Why not let the world serve as an external memory, as O'Regan (1992) has argued, or why not let the world serve, in Brooks's (1991) phrase, as its own model?[14] It makes good evolutionary and engineering sense to *off-load* the representations. We are built in such a way that we can get the information about the world that we need, when we need it.

The claim is not that there are no representations in vision. That is a strong claim that most cognitive scientists would reject. The claim rather is that the role of representations in perceptual theory needs to be reconsidered. (See Noë, Pessoa, and Thompson 2000; Noë 2001; O'Regan and Noë 2001a.) It is a mistake to suppose that vision just is a process whereby an internal world-model is built up, and that the task-level characterization of vision (what Marr [1982, 23–31] called the computational theory of vision) should treat vision as a process whereby a unified internal model of the world is generated. This is compatible with there being all sorts of representations in the brain, and indeed, with the presence of such representations being necessary for perception.[15] Marr famously claimed of

Gibson that he "vastly underrated the sheer difficulty" of the information-processing problem of vision (1982, 30). As the vision scientist Nakayama has responded (1994), there's reason to think that Marr and his followers underestimated the difficulty of correctly framing what vision is at the task or computational level. Vision isn't a process whereby the brain constructs a detailed internal world representation. Once one acknowledges this, then "detailed internal world representations" can be demoted from their theoretical pride of place.

I have argued that the role of representations in perceptual theory needs to be reconsidered. (See Noë, Pessoa, and Thompson 2000; Noë 2001a; O'Regan and Noë 2001a.) This is exactly the path explored by Dana Ballard's animate vision program (Ballard 1991, 1996, 2002). To understand his approach, suppose you are in strange city and your task is to reach the castle on the hill in the center of town. Compare two possible strategies. On a first strategy, you make use of a map. You plot your position on the map, and that of the castle, and you figure out a path connecting the two points. Now you're ready to roll. As you move along, you keep track of your progress on the map. If the map's a good one—if there is a one-to-one correspondence between points in space, and points on the map, and if you don't get confused about what you're doing, you'll get to your goal.

The second strategy is simpler, and somewhat cruder. You look around and notice that you can see the castle on the hill. You can see it rising up on a ridge on the other side of town. So you dispense with a map and head out in the direction of the castle. You just keep the castle locked into view. This second strategy may be crude, but it has distinct advantages. For one thing, to pursue it you don't need a map. Maps are expensive and they are not all that easy to use. It takes time to study the map, to pinpoint yourself and your goal, and so forth. But there is a downside too. The strategy will only work if you can actually see the target (if your eyes are good, if it isn't night), and if heading toward it is likely to reveal a path leading up to it. In a maze-like city, where many ways dead-end, and others lead around the mountain, not up it, the second strategy won't work. That it works depends on the way the environment is, on your skills, and on the way you are embedded in that environment.

Ballard, who works in robotics and artificial intelligence, has proposed that given the nature of our environment, and the way we are embedded in it, vision is in a position to take advantage of something like the second strategy. Traditional approaches to vision have always assumed that we deploy the first strategy. If your aim is to pick up a coffee cup, reasons Ballard, you don't need *first* to build up a detailed internal representation of the cup in space (Ballard 1996). You can just lock your gaze on the cup—your gaze is a way of pointing at the cup, a *deictic* act—and let the cup play a role in guiding your hand to it. Instead of plotting a course through an internal map, you act on what you look at, and you let the fact that what interests you is there in front of you play a guiding function. An important consequence of this proposal is that it lessens the representational burden of the system, and that it does so by making explicit use of our bodily skills. Instead of having to ground ourselves by sheer cognition—constructing a representation of the point in space in our minds—we take advantage of the fact that we have more immediate links to the world because we are in the world from the start, and that we have the sorts of bodily skills to exploit those linkages.[16]

1.6   Persons and Their Bodies

The computational theory of vision stakes itself on the claim that what Marr called the algorithmic level of description of cognitive phenomena is autonomous with respect to the implementational level. Low-level, concrete facts about the brain and nervous system may be constraints on the processes unfolding at the higher level. But crucially, the transactions of the higher level are independent of what goes on at the lower level in both a metaphysical and an epistemological sense. Metaphysically, they are independent in that they are not constituted by what happens at the implementational level. So, for example, one and the same algorithmic system could be implemented by different physical systems. Epistemologically, they are independent in that one can fully understand the algorithmic processes without understanding how they are implemented. These metaphysical and epistemological factors gain support from methodological considerations as well. Marr thought that you couldn't develop a sound theory of vision from the bottom up. He wrote, "Trying to understand vision by studying only neurons is like trying to understand bird flight by studying only feathers: It just cannot be done" (Marr 1982, 27). The guiding metaphor is familiar: Psychology studies cognitive processes at a more abstract level than that of their biological realization just as the programmer studies computational processes at a more abstract level than that of their realization in the hardware of the machine.

A lot is supposed to hang on this autonomy of levels. For one thing, it is supposed to explain how a materialist can insist that psychology has a special domain of inquiry different from that of brain science (Fodor 1975; Dennett [1981] 1987). Psychology is interested in what the brain does, but at higher levels of abstraction than that of neuroscience. It is precisely this autonomy of levels that enabled Chomsky (e.g., 1965, 1980) to claim that linguistic theory seeks to explore language as part of our biological endowment, but in a manner completely divorced from the study of linguistic performance, on the one hand, or biological realization in the brain, on the other.

The enactive view applies pressure to the autonomy thesis. If perception is in part constituted by our possession and exercise of bodily skills—as I argue in this book—then it may also depend on our possession of the sort of bodies that can encompass those skills, for only a creature with such a body could have those skills. To perceive like us, it follows, you must have a body like ours. In general it is a mistake to think that we can sharply distinguish visual processing at the highly abstract algorithmic level, on the one hand, from processing at the concrete implementational level, on the other. The point is not that algorithms are constrained by their implementation, although that is true. The point, rather, is that the algorithms are actually, at least in part, formulated *in terms of* items at the implementational level. You might actually need to mention hands and eyes in the algorithms!

As an illustration, consider that, according to the enactive approach, vision depends on one's knowledge of the sensory effects of, say, eye movements, for example, movements of the eye to the right causes a shift to the left in the retinal image. This knowledge is eye-dependent. Or consider a different kind of case. We noted above that Ballard proposes that the perceptual localization of an object, such as a cup on the table before us, may depend on the gaze-fixing mechanisms of the eye. The algorithm says "reach where I'm looking now" or "put your hand here now" rather than something like "the cup is at such and such a point in space; move your hand there." Space may be represented not absolutely, but rather precisely in terms of movements. In this way, eyes, hands, and the neural systems

that enable eye and hand movements are not merely ways of implemen-
ting a spatial perception and action algorithm, they are elements in the
computations themselves.

A phenomenological example can help illustrate the way our bodies can
enter into our experience. Suppose you are in an airplane. At takeoff it will
look to you as if the front of the plane, the nose, rises or lifts up in your
field of vision. In fact, it does not. Because you move with the plane, the
nose of the plane does not lift relative to you. No lifting, strictly speaking,
is visible from where you sit. What explains the illusion of the apparent rising of the nose? When the plane rises, your vestibular system detects your
movement relative to the direction of gravity. This causes it to look to you
as if the nose is rising.[17] The nose is rising, and it looks to you as if it is.
But not for visual reasons. This phenomenon illustrates, first, one of the
errors implicit in the idea of Pure Vision. How things are experienced *visually* depends on more than merely optical processes. This is a respect in
which the content of a visual experience is not like the content of a photograph. Second, the example illustrates the way in which the character of our
visual experience depends on our embodiment, that is, on idiosyncratic
aspects of our sensory implementation.

I have said that only a creature with a body like ours can have experiences like ours. But now we ask: Must a creature have a body *exactly* like
ours to have experience enough like ours to be thought of as *perceptual*, say,
or as *visual*? That would be an undesirable consequence, ruling out even a
very weak multiple realizability of sensory systems.[18] Clark and Toribio
(2001; Clark 2002) have suggested that the enactive approach has this consequence, and that, therefore, the view is guilty of a kind of "sensorimotor
chauvinism."

To respond to this, consider Bach-y-Rita's prosthetic visual system
known as the tactile-vision substitution system (TVSS) (1972, 1983, 1984,
1996). Visual stimulation received by a head-mounted camera is trans-
duced to activate an array of vibrators on the thigh of a blind subject. If
the subject is free to move around and thus control tactile-motor dependencies, after a time she reports that she has the experience of objects
arrayed in three-dimensional space. She is able to make judgments about
the number, relative size, and position of objects in the environment. This
is a mode of prosthetic perception. Crucially, it is not a mode of perception
by touch, despite the fact that it enables the subject to perceive thanks to

the activation of sensory receptors in the skin and neural processes in the somatosensory cortex. For touch is a way of perceiving by bringing things up against you, into contact with your skin. It is reasonable to admit that the resulting experiences are, if not fully visual, then vision-like to some extent. For example, using TVSS subjects describe objects being blocked from view when an opaque object interposes, and subjects are unable to perceive using TVSS if the lights are turned off. So let us say, then, that TVSS enables a kind of tactile vision. This is seeing (or quasi-seeing) without the deployment of the parts of body and brain normally dedicated to seeing, for example, the eyes and visual cortex. This is a striking example of multiple realization and neural plasticity. Somatosensory neural activity realizes visual experiences.[19]

The existence of tactile vision and related forms of sensory substitution provides strong support for the enactive view. As O'Regan and I have argued, they provide evidence for the view because they illustrate that perceptual experience depends constitutively on the exercise of sensorimotor knowledge (O'Regan and Noë 2001a,b; Noë 2002a; see also Hurley and Noë 2003a,b). Tactile vision is vision-like because (or to the extent that) there is, as it were, an isomorphism at the sensorimotor level between tactile vision and normal vision. In tactile vision, movements with respect to the environment produce changes in stimulation that are similar in pattern to those encountered during normal vision. The same reservoir of sensorimotor skill is drawn on in both instances.

The enactive view, in turn, exhibits the sort of principles of embodiment that place constraints on what degrees of similarity of body are required to achieve similarity of experience. Tactile vision is vision-like to the extent that there exists a sensorimotor isomorphism between vision and tactile vision. But tactile vision is unlike vision precisely to the extent that this sensorimotor isomorphism fails to obtain. It will fail to obtain, in general, whenever the two candidate realizing systems differ in what we can think of as their sensorimotor multiplicity (i.e., in their ability to subserve patterns of sensorimotor dependence). TVSS and the human visual system are very different in respect to their sensorimotor multiplicity. Compare the crudity and simplicity of the vibrator array in TVSS with the refinement and complexity of the retina. Only a vibrator array with something like the functional multiplicity of the retina could support genuine (full-fledged, normal) vision. To make tactile vision *more* fully visual, then, we need to make the physical system on which it depends more like the human visual system.

In this way, the charge of sensorimotor chauvinism can be answered. Insofar as the enactive approach is willing to count TVSS as quasi-visual, the charge of chauvinism can hardly be made to stick. Nevertheless, differences in body make for differences in sensorimotor skills and in experience. It is not chauvinism to recognize that there will be qualitative differences between TVSS and vision owing to the different ways these systems are embodied.

1.7 A Psychology of the Personal Level?

There is a further enactive challenge to the computer model of mind. Computational theories of vision, for example, model vision as a computation implemented in the brain. Such theories attempt to explain, in the domain of vision, how the brain, which is merely a "syntactic engine," can come to function as a "semantic engine," that is, how it can, for example, produce a detailed representation of the scene on the basis of meaningless patterns of light hitting nerve endings (Dennett [1981] 1987). As Dennett ([1978] 1981) has argued, one of the chief fruits of the computational approach, as a framework for philosophical and empirical investigation of mind, is that it provides, or at least seems to provide, an account of how the brain performs these computational functions, and it does so in a way that satisfies two apparently incompatible desiderata. First, the computational approach explains how the brain gives rise to perception, but it does so not in the idiom of neuroscience (e.g., in terms of action potentials, etc.), but rather in the apparently personal-level idiom of intentional ascription (e.g., in terms of signaling, representing, inferring, guessing, etc.). Second, the computational approach manages to satisfy the first desideratum *without* committing the homunculus fallacy (Kenny 1971 [1984], 1989; Searle 1992; Bennett and Hacker 2001). How is the computational approach supposed to achieve this?

The point of the first desideratum is clear. The alternative to deploying a richly intentional idiom to explain what the brain does, in Dennett's words, "is not really psychology at all, but just at best abstract neurophysiology—pure internal syntax with no hope of semantic interpretation. Psychology 'reduced' to neurophysiology in this fashion would not be psychology, for it would not be able to provide an explanation of the regularities it is psychology's particular job to explain: The reliability with which 'intelligent' organisms can cope with their environments and thus prolong their lives" ([1978] 1987, 64). The point of the second desideratum is equally clear. We won't have succeeded in explaining anything if, in describing the brain in an intentional idiom, we tacitly assume that the subsystems of the brain have the very cognitive powers we are seeking to explain. The solution, according to Dennett, is the insistence that we do not suppose that the internal subsystems have the very powers we seek to explain. Rather, we suppose that they have powers like ours, but simpler. The intuition is that we can decompose the system into homunculi whose powers are so simple as to be, plausibly, powers of the neurons themselves.

Searle has criticized this account of the foundations of the computational theory on the grounds that it confuses the claim that the lowest level of homunculi perform *very simple* functions with the claim that they perform *semantically innocent* functions (Searle 1992). Insofar as we view these maximally simple homunculi as performing functions of symbolic significance, then there's nothing semantically innocent about them.

Whether or not we find Searle's criticism plausible, it seems that from the standpoint of the enactive view at least (which is not Searle's standpoint), Dennett's proposed solution may not avail. Dennett argues that we can explain the brain's semantic powers without attributing non-dischargable semantic powers to the brain's subsystems. But according to the enactive view, perception isn't something that unfolds in the brain *however characterized*, whether in information-processing terms, or those of neurophysiology. It is not the brain, it is the animal (or person), who sees. It's the person, not the brain, that has semantic powers. In a sense, then, the homuncular decomposition never succeeds in discharging the biggest subpersonal homunculus of them all—namely, the brain itself—for the computational approach never allows us to discharge—or better, free ourselves from—the idea that we are analyzing the semantic powers of the brain.

I take it that this is the significance of Nakayama's (1994) remark, mentioned earlier, regarding Marr's oversimplification of the computational problem of vision. Vision shouldn't be thought of as a computation performed by the brain on inputs provided by the retina. What is vision? How should it be characterized computationally? This book suggests the outlines of an answer. *Vision is a mode of exploration of the environment drawing on implicit understanding of sensorimotor regularities* (O'Regan and Noë 2001a,b). To model vision correctly, then, we must model it not as something that takes place inside the animal's brain, but as something that directly involves not only the brain but also the animate body and the world.

I have been making use of Dennett's distinction between the personal and the subpersonal (Dennett 1969). But it now appears that we cannot make quite the same use of the distinction that McDowell (1994b) and others have suggested. McDowell sought to reconcile Gibsonian and computational approaches to vision by suggesting that the former provides a theory of vision *at the personal level*, while Marr and the computationalists are concerned with modeling subpersonal processes, that is, the processes that causally underpin and enable the person to see. The flaw in this proposed rapprochement is this: If Gibson is right that the subject of perception is the whole animal, actively exploring its environment, then Marr's characterization of vision at the subpersonal level must be wrongheaded, for he characterizes the subpersonal processes not merely as contributing to the enabling of seeing, but as constituting seeing itself.

The upshot of these reflections, however, is not that we need a theory of perception at the personal level. Dennett insists that this can't be done and he suggests that Ryle, Wittgenstein, and Gibson are *anti-science* in the end because they insist that the only satisfactory account must be at the personal level. Whether or not this is right, I am now inclined to agree with Fodor that the distinction between the person and the subpersonal causal processes enabling mental life may not matter for cognitive science, or may not matter nearly as much as McDowell and others have thought: "Whatever the relevance the distinction between states of the organism and states of its nervous system may have for *some* purposes, there is no particular reason to suppose that it is relevant to the purposes of cognitive psychology" (Fodor 1975, 52). The reason for this is that it turns out that it's not possible to draw a sharp line between what is done by the person, or animal, and what is done by the subpersonal system, or by parts of the animal. This is not to say that there are no straightforward cases. I see. My heart pounds. *I* don't pound my heart. On the other hand, some of the time when my eyes move, it is I who move them, and very often, even if I am not directing their movements, I make use of their movements to keep track of what's going on around me. When my eyes move, whether they move as a result of volition or not, they give rise to changes, some of which (changes in how things look) I may be aware of, and others of which (changes in patterns of retinal activity) I am not. Yet even the subconscious changes (subconscious because subpersonal) may matter to me and impinge on my awareness. As a perceiver I understand, implicitly, how to modulate them. For example, when I cup my ears to hear something better, I modulate receptor-level events to which I have no direct access. But I cup my ears precisely in order to do this, that is, to increase the intensity of stimulation in my ears. Consider the pounding of my heart again. If I am a long-distance runner, then I am used to a certain kind of increased level of pounding. If my heart were to pound that way when I was at rest though, that would be alarming. The point is, as a runner, I have some degree of access to, and control over, subpersonal processes within me. To some extent, my skills as a runner comprise the ability to make my body do this and that. In general, I depend on my subpersonal parts, not merely causally, but constitutively. For I am—we are—beings whose minds are shaped by a complicated hierarchy of practical skills. Our consciousness frequently does not extend to what is going on in our bodies; our consciousness is enacted by what we do with our bodies.

This is not to deny that a distinction can be drawn between the personal and the subpersonal. When I attribute a psychological state to you, it is plausible that I view you as subject to, as it is said, normative constraints of rationality and the holism of the mental. Only a person with a modicum of rationality and a wealth of background knowledge can have, for example, the thought that he or she would like to be rich. And when I attribute to your brain a certain level of activity (say, on the basis of a functional magnetic resonance imagery [fMRI] scan), I do so without regard to such constraints. What you believe or want or expect has no bearing on my attribution of blood-flow activity to your brain on the basis of fMRI.

The understanding of concepts is usually supposed to be a paradigm of personal-level accomplishment. But just as there is no sharp line between the personal and the subpersonal, so there may be no sharp line between the conceptual and the nonconceptual. Indeed, it may be that sensorimotor skills deserve to be thought of as primitive conceptual skills, even if, as is frequently the case, they are subpersonal. I take this up again in chapter 6.

For these reasons, it seems, a theory of perception must straddle the divide between the personal and subpersonal, just as it must straddle the divide between what is conscious and what is unconscious, and what is conceptual and what is nonconceptual. What will such a theory look like? This book is meant to be a step toward an answer.

1.8 Behaviorism Revisited?

I conclude this chapter by considering an objection that may have occurred to the reader. Isn't the kind of identification of perception and action that gets made in this book a form of behaviorism? Experience is *not* something we do; it is something we undergo, something that happens in us! Block (2001), for example, has argued that O'Regan and I are behaviorists because we hold that to have an experience is to partake in certain patterns of input-output relations.

In order to answer this charge, let's consider a different kind of example.

Suppose you hear me say: "Nein!" How do you experience what I say? If you know German, and if the context is right, you may experience me as saying the German word for "No." If you do not know German, but only English, and if the context is different, you may understand me as saying the English word for the number 9. Depending on what you know, and depending on the context, one and the same accoustic phenomenon will lead to very different experiences in you. How you experience my utterance depends not on what you do, but on what knowledge you bring to bear in "making sense" of the stimulus. It is of course true that, given what you know and what knowledge you make use of, your experience of understanding me will dispose you to act in different ways. You will be disposed to reply in some way or other, for example, and the character of your disposition will differ depending on your experience. But it would be a mistake, I think, to say that your experiencing the word one way or the other is simply a matter of your different dispositions. That is the mistake of behaviorism.

According to the enactive approach to perceptual experience, there is all the difference in the world between experiencing the red of a flower, or the shape of a sculpture, and merely having behavioral dispositions. How you experience the flower or the sculpture depends on your perceptual knowledge and on the skill with which you bring this knowledge to bear on what you encounter. As in the linguistic case described earlier, the behaviorist is right that to differences in experiences there correspond differences in behavioral dispositions (other things being equal). But from this it doesn't follow that there is no experience. The enactive view certainly does not embrace the behaviorist's denial of experience. Far from it. As we will see, one of the central aims of this book is to investigate the phenomenology of perceptual experience.

As O'Regan and I stressed in our (2001b) reply to Block, the key to our theory is the idea that perception depends on the possession and exercise of a certain kind of practical knowledge. This is not a behaviorist thesis.[20]

1.9   The Book in Outline

I propose that to perceive is not merely to have sensation, or to receive sensory impressions, it is to have sensations that one understands. The aim of this book is to investigate the forms this understanding can take. There are two main kinds here, although, as I have indicated, there may be no sharp line to be drawn between them. First, there is sensorimotor understanding. Second, there is conceptual understanding. I have said little about the second kind so far. I turn to a discussion of it in chapter 6.

The main argument begins in chapter 2, whose topic is the phenomenology of perception. I argue, on phenomenological grounds, that the content of perception is not like the content of a picture. In particular, the detailed world is not given to consciousness all at once in the way detail is contained in a picture. In vision, as in touch, we gain perceptual content by active inquiry and exploration. When we see, for example, we are not aware of the whole scene in all its detail all at once. We do enjoy a sense of the presence of a whole detailed scene, but it is no part of our phenomenology that the experience represents all the detail all at once in consciousness. The detail is experienced by us as *out there*, not as *in our minds*.

This gives rise to a puzzle. How can we explain our sense, now, of the presence of the whole scene, if we do not actually represent the scene now in full detail the way a picture does? In what does our sense of perceptual contact with the dense and detailed environment consist? I call this the puzzle of perceptual presence. In the course of developing a solution to this proposal, I lay out the enactive (what O'Regan and I have called the sensorimotor) approach to perception. I argue, in particular, that our sense of the presence of detail is to be understood in terms of our *access* to detail thanks to our possession of sensorimotor skill.

The heart of the book is chapters 3 and 4. In these chapters I argue that perceptual experience acquires content thanks to our possession and exercise of practical bodily knowledge. In chapter 3 I focus on the problem of spatial content. The focus of chapter 4 is the experience of color.

In chapter 5, I consider the so-called causal theory of perception. This is a theory of the role of *causation in perception*. I try to show that by emphasizing the role of *action in perception*, the causal theory can overcome important obstacles. But the more far-reaching conclusion of this chapter is that what philosophers call the representational content of experience must be understood to include a *perspectival* aspect. This perspectival aspect marks the place of action in perception. To perceive, we need to keep track of our movements relative to the world. This perspectival aspect belongs to what is experienced.

Perceptual experience is radically ambiguous. The question *What do we experience?* always admits different answers. When we see, we see both how things are, and also how they appear to be. But these are not always the same. For example, we see that the plate is circular, and that it looks elliptical from here. This ambiguity is the source of two important puzzles in the theory of perception, one philosophical and the other psychological. The psychological puzzle is that of perceptual constancy—that is, the phenomenon exemplified by such a fact as that then when you take a book outdoors it does not appear to change color even though the character or the light it reflects changes radically. The philosophical puzzle is that of direct perception, that is, whether the direct objects of perception are mental items such as "sense data." These are puzzles about perceptual content. In chapter 6 I suggest that their solution may turn on an assessment of the place of thought in experience.

Chapter 7 takes up the question of perceptual experience and the brain. In this final chapter I explore the implications of the enactive approach for understanding the brain basis of perceptual consciousness.

2 Pictures in Mind

The eye is not a camera that forms and delivers an image, nor is the retina simply a keyboard that can be struck by fingers of light.
—J. J. Gibson

Vision is a palpation with the look.
—M. Merleau-Ponty

2.1 The Snapshot Conception

When we try to understand the nature of sensory perception, we tend to think in terms of vision, and when we think of vision, we tend to suppose that the eye is like a camera and that vision is a quasi-photographic process. To see, we suppose, is to undergo snapshot-like experiences of the scene before us. You open your eyes and you are given experiences that represent the scene—picture-like—in sharp focus and uniform detail from the center out to the periphery.

This snapshot conception of visual experience is neatly captured by Mach's famous drawing of the visual field (Mach [1886] 1959). Mach's drawing (see figure 2.1), is not meant to be a picture of the room, or even a picture of the room as seen from a particular point of view (reclining on a divan, with right eye shut, fixating a point straight ahead). Rather, it is meant to be a depiction of what the seeing of the room is like, a treatment of the visual experience itself. Mach's drawing represents visual experience as sharply focused, uniformly detailed, and high-resolution. The visible world is represented in consciousness in full detail.[1]

Something like the snapshot conception provides the starting point for much empirical work on vision. The basic problem that vision science

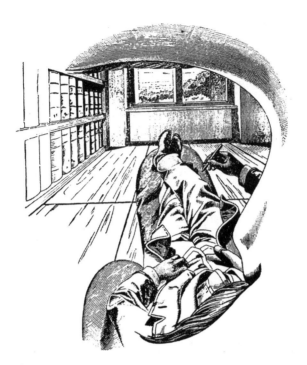

Figure 2.1
Mach's picture of the visual field (from Mach [1886] 1959).

faces (at least as it has been conceived over the last century and a half) is that of explaining how it is that we can enjoy this sort of richly detailed, high-resolution visual experience, when our actual perceptual contact with the world, in the form of the stimulation of the retina, is so limited. The psychologist Richard Gregory puts the problem like this: "We are given tiny distorted upside-down images in the eye, and we see solid objects in surrounding space. From patterns of stimulation on the retinas we perceive the world of objects, and this is nothing short of a miracle" ([1966] 1997, 9). The fundamental problem for visual science has been to understand how the brain performs this miracle. Or perhaps we should say, it has been to understand how it can be that it isn't really a miracle at all.

The challenge is even greater than Gregory indicates. There is an enormous discrepancy between the character of the input to vision—Gregory's tiny, distorted, upside-down retinal images—and the high-resolution colorful world that we know in experience. The fundamental problem for visual theory is to understand how the brain makes up for this discrepancy.

As an example, consider the fact that the eye is in nearly constant motion, saccading two or three times a second. Because of this, the retinal image is in nearly constant motion relative to the eye. How is it then that we perceive the world as generally stable? The problem is quite thorny. Consider that when you track a moving object with your eyes, the image of the object itself is relatively stable on the eye; after all, the eye moves with the object. The background against which the object is perceived as moving, in contrast, which is perceived as still, literally races across the eye (as discussed in Bridgeman, Van der Heijden, and Velichkovsky 1994). Somehow, it would seem, the brain must distinguish between the movement of the retinal image, on the one hand, and the movement of things in the world, on the other.[2] According to what we can think of as the orthodox approach to visual perception, the brain must then construct a representation of what is seen that compensates for movements of the retinal image itself.[3] This is a striking example of the way visual theory seeks to make up for a discrepancy between the character of the retinal image and the content of perceptual experience; somehow the brain must bridge the gap.

There are numerous other respects in which the retinal picture can be thought of as distorted or defective. Blood vessels and nerve fibers are positioned *in front of* the receptors on the retina. These obstructions block and refract incoming light, and they cast shadows. In addition, the eye's resolving power is nonuniform. Rods and cones are not evenly distributed across the surface of the retina. Outside the high-resolution central (foveal) region, there are increasingly few cones. As a result of this, the eye is nearly color-blind in its parafoveal region. Despite these "defects," we do not experience the world, so to speak, as black-and-white at the edges. But shouldn't we? The orthodox proposal is that the brain produces an improved representation in which these limitations of the retinal image have been corrected. Our experience is that of a uniformly colorful world in Machian detail because the representation that actually forms the substrate of our experience represents the world in high-resolution color, unlike the retinal image on the basis of which it is constructed.

The idea that vision is a process of correcting for imperfections in the retinal image is beautifully illustrated by a consideration of the so-called optic disk. In each retina there is a small region where there are no photoreceptors. This is where axons from retinal ganglion cells come together to form the optic nerve. As a result of this "blind spot" there is, in some sense, a gap or discontinuity in the retinal image. There is, of course, no corresponding gap or discontinuity in our visual experience. How does the brain make up for this discrepancy between what is given to us in the retinal image and what is experienced? To some extent, we can explain our failure to notice a gap by the fact that what falls on the blind spot of one eye does not fall on the blind spot of the other eye, and by the fact that the eyes are in nearly constant motion so that what falls on the blind spot now may not a moment later. However we do not experience a hole in the visual field even when we use only one eye. How is this to be explained?

Many scientists conclude that the brain *fills in* the gap in the internal representation of the scene. How else can we explain the fact that, as vision scientist Stephen Palmer writes, "We fail to experience any sensory gap at the blind spot" (1999a, 617)? Palmer goes on to state that we *know* that the sensory gap is filled in thanks to the results of demonstrations such as that given in figure 2.2. Shut your right eye and fixate on the cross with your left eye. Adjust the distance of the book from your eye. At one point (when the page is about 8 to 12 inches from your face) the gap in the line on the right falls within the blind spot. What do we experience when that happens? When the gap falls on the blind spot, it looks as if the line is solid. The gap is literally filled in in our experience. As Palmer writes, "The line on the retina actually has a gap in it at the blind spot, but we experience it as complete and uninterrupted when the gap falls within the blind spot. The important point is that what we experience visually conforms not to the firing of retinal receptors, but to some higher level of neural activity" (1999a, 617). Neural processes of filling in a higher-level neural representation are what bridge the gap between low-level retinal input and experience.

Orthodox visual theory in this way frames its central problem as that of constructing an internal representation sufficient to support our detailed,

Figure 2.2
Filling in at the blind spot: Shut your right eye and fixate the cross with your left. Adjust the distance of the book from your eye. At one point the gap in the line on the right falls within the so-called blind spot. What do you experience when that happens?

high-resolution, gap-free, snapshot-like (Machian) visual experiences of the world despite the imperfections and limitations of the retinal image itself. The theory of vision, according to this orthodox standpoint, is the theory of the ways the brain corrects for and overcomes these limitations.

2.2   Fallacies Pictorial and Homuncular

The snapshot conception is an idea about the phenomenology of visual experience, about what seeing is like. Seeing the world, so the conception would have it, is like having detailed pictures of the world in mind. Visual experiences represent the world the way pictures do, in sharp focus and uniform detail. My main aim in this chapter is to explore, and reject, this way of thinking about the character of experience.

But first let's consider two further, related ideas about the pictorial character of seeing. First, there is the idea that the basis (the input) for vision is a picture, the *retinal* picture. In this vein, David Marr wrote that vision "is the process of discovering *from images* what is present in the world, and where it is" (Marr 1982, 3, my italics). Presumably the images he had in mind were those projected onto the retina. Seeing depends on retinal pictures. Second, there is the idea we have just considered (in section 2.1) that vision is a process whereby the brain, starting from the retinal picture, produces a better, more detailed neural picture or representation. This is nicely illustrated by the example of filling in at the blind spot. To explain the fact that we do not experience a gap in the visual field, it is supposed that the brain fills in the discontinuity in the retinal image; it produces a gap-free picture that can then serve as the internal substrate of our gap-free experience of the world.[4]

These further ideas about the role of pictures in vision are strictly independent of the snapshot conception. One might hold that vision relies on pictures in these ways even if the content of perceptual experience is not picture-like. And one could hold to the snapshot conception without believing that the causal mechanisms underlying visual experience requires pictures in just the way the orthodox conception seems to suppose. (This is an important point to which I will return.) Nevertheless, these three general ideas about the pictorial character of vision—that vision starts with retinal pictures that are transformed into better internal pictures that give rise to experiences with picture-like content—are related just as the members of a family are related. They have grown up together and they are mutually supporting. As we have noticed, the central problem orthodox visual theory faces is that of explaining how we can have the sort of picture-like experience the snapshot conception says we enjoy when the content of the retinal picture falls so far short of the content of our experience. It is perhaps a natural further step to suppose that our experience is picture-like *because* we experience what is represented by a picture in the head, a picture that is constructed from the starting point of the retinal picture.

The idea that vision is, in these ways, a pictorial process has ancient roots. Leonardo da Vinci compared the eye to a pinhole camera (a *camera obscura*).[5] Kepler later demonstrated that the eye's optics are such that light striking the eye is refracted by the cornea and brought to a focus so as to produce an actual picture on the retina. In this way he showed that the eye is very literally a device for making pictures. He wrote: "Thus vision is brought about by a picture of the thing seen being formed on the concave surface of the retina . . . the greater the acuity of vision of a given person, the finer will be the picture formed in his eye" (Kepler [1951] 1964, 150, quoted in Wade 1998, 9). A few years later, Scheiner (1619) showed how, it is possible actually to *see* the retinal picture in an excised animal's eye (as reported in Wade 1998, 26).[6] The basic idea has been illustrated by Descartes (see figure 2.3).

A brief sketch of some of the background history of debates in this area is telling.[7] The pictorial approach has not always seemed so natural. Euclid and Ptolemy had endorsed Plato's idea that when we see, visual rays shoot forth from the eye and so bring us into contact with objects (1929 *Timaeus*, 45b–d).[8] This *extromissionist* theory of vision laid the groundwork for mathematical optics;[9] in practice the visual rays could be treated as geometrical lines; by their means it is possible to model the geometry of our visual relation to the environment.

Aristotle rejected this Platonic extromissionism in favor of an *intromissionist* view. But his theory was no more pictorial than Euclid and Ptolemy's. Seeing, according to Aristotle, is a process whereby the *form* of an object but not its matter enters into the eye.[10] This makes intuitive sense: The roundness of the object, say, but not the object itself enters into the eye and so affects our "common sense."

But Aristotle's intromissionism has shortcomings from which the Platonic view did not suffer. As Al-Kindi argued in the ninth century, Aristotle's

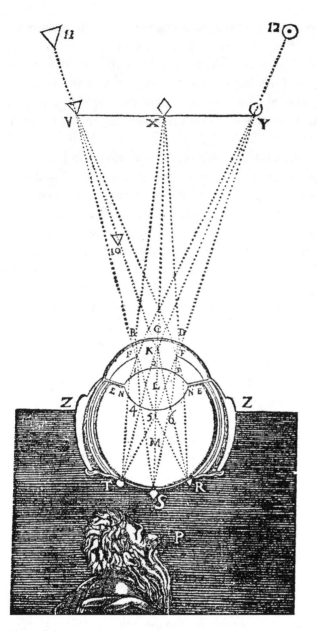

Figure 2.3
Descartes' illustration of the theory of the retinal image from his *La Dioptrique*
([1637] 1902), after Lindberg 1976, 201.

transmission-of-forms view fails to do justice to perspective in visual experience.[11] The form of the plate may be circular. But surely when you see a plate from an angle, it does not look circular, but rather elliptical. Since seeing the plate from a particular angle is, according to Aristotle, the act of receiving its one and only form (without the matter), the plate ought to look the same from any vantage point if this theory is right. Of course it does not.

The tenth-century Arab theorist Alhazen (Ibn Haythem) sought to combine the Aristotelian idea that when we see, forms enter the eye, with the Platonic mathematical theory of rays.[12] Aware of Al-Kindi's criticism of Aristotle, Alhazen provided a geometrical reinterpretation of Aristotle's transmission of forms. Alhazen gives meaning to the Aristotelian theory that sight involves the receiving of forms of objects, by treating the forms that are transmitted as images in the mathematical (but not in the pictorial) sense.[13] In this way Alhazen reinterprets the Aristotelian idea of form in a way that makes it amenable to geometrical analysis. He does so in a way that handles Al-Kindi's criticism of the transmission-of-forms view. The form of a plate seen at an angle, in this view, is different from that of a plate seen from straight on.[14]

Enter Kepler: Kepler's contribution was, in effect, to refine Alhazen's theory against the background of a better understanding of the anatomy and optics of the eye.[15] Kepler showed that the rays of light entering the eye are brought to a focus on the back of the eye in such a way as to give rise not merely to an image in the mathematical sense, but to a genuinely *pictorial* image. The eye functions as a *true* picture-making machine. Aristotle's forms become actual pictures on the eye. Descartes' illustration (figure 2.3) serves as an adequate representation of Kepler's theory of the retinal image.[16]

It is to Kepler, then, that we owe the idea that seeing depends on the existence of pictures in the eye. Insofar as this idea has driven the modern study of vision, Kepler deserves to be thought of as the founder of the modern theory of vision. But it is striking that Kepler's view is really the culmination of a medieval debate, rather than the start of a whole new way of thinking about the nature of vision.

The theory of the retinal picture gives rise to puzzles of its own. First, there is the problem of the inverted image. How is it that we see the world upright, when the retinal image is upside down? Second, there is the problem of "cyclopean" vision. There are *two*, slightly different retinal images. How is it that we enjoy a single, unified visual experience of the world? Theorists today are still moved by these two puzzles, even though very few of them would admit it. Gregory, for example, in the passage cited earlier, calls attention to the fact that the two images in the eyes are upside down; he does this precisely in order to explain what I have called the fundamental problem of vision. Pinker, in a recent survey of visual theory, writes that "many kinds of animals have two eyes, and whenever they aim forward, so that their fields overlap (rather than aiming outward for a panoramic view) natural selection must have faced the problem of combining their pictures into a unified image that the rest of the brain can use" (1997, 218).

Kepler "tortured himself" trying to solve the problem of the inverted image.[17] Because projective geometry dictates that the image is inverted when it enters the eye, Kepler explored whether the image is reinverted before landing on the retina. Leonardo also seems to have supposed that there is need for a reinversion. This supposition is captured in figure 2.4.[18]

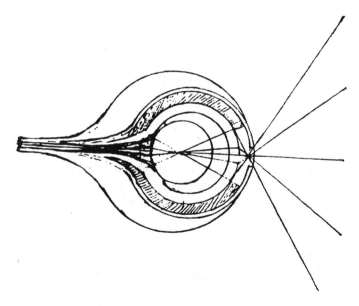

Figure 2.4
Leonardo's representation of upright vision (c. 1500) as resulting from an optical reinversion, from Wade 1998, 323.

In the end Kepler seems to have settled on the idea that the resolution of this problem lies outside the sphere of optics, which is concerned primarily with geometrical laws. Kepler writes:

I say that vision occurs when the image of the whole hemisphere of the world that is before the eye . . . is fixed on the reddish white concave surface of the retina. How the image or picture is composed by the visual spirits that reside in the retina and the [optic] nerve, and whether it is made to appear before the soul or the tribunal of the visual faculty by a spirit within the hollows of the brain, or whether the visual faculty, like a magistrate sent by the soul, goes forth from the administrative chamber of the brain into the optic nerve and the retina to meet this image, as though descending to a lower court—[all] this I leave to be disputed by the physicists. For the armament of the opticians does not take them beyond this first opaque wall encountered within the eye. (qtd. in Lindberg 1976, 203)

The first thinker to find a clear path through this thicket of puzzles about the retinal image was Descartes. He believed that the problem of the inverted retinal image is an artifact of dubious assumptions and is, in this sense, a pseudoproblem. He argued that it is not as a *picture* that the retinal image figures in a causal, mechanical account of vision. It "is necessary to beware of assuming," he wrote, "that in order to sense, the mind needs to perceive certain images transmitted by the objects to the brain, as our philosophers commonly suppose" (Descartes [1637] 1965, 89). It is rather only insofar as the picture is composed of movements, which it transmits along the nerves to the brain, that the retinal images are necessary for vision. He wrote:

Now although this picture, in being so transmitted into our head, always retains some resemblance to the objects from which it proceeds, nevertheless, as I have already shown, we must not hold that it is by means of this resemblance that the picture causes us to perceive the objects, as if there were yet other eyes in our brain with which we could apprehend it; but rather, that it is the movements of which the picture is composed which, acting immediately on our mind inasmuch as it is united to our body, are so established by nature as to make it have such perceptions. (Descartes [1637] 1965, 101)

In these passages Descartes spells out what has since come to be known as the homunculus fallacy, or the fallacy of the little man in the head (Kenny [1971] 1994; Dennett [1978] 1981; Searle 1992; Bennett and Hacker 2001). It is incoherent to suppose that seeing an object depends on the resemblance between a picture in the eye and the object, for that presupposes that there is, as it were, someone inside the head who perceives the resemblance. This would lead to a regress, as there is no less diffi-culty explaining how the interior observer can see the interior picture. The source of the fallacy of the little man in the head is the idea that the retinal picture functions as a picture, as something *perceived*.

If the retinal image does not function as a picture in producing vision, then it must function in some other way. Descartes proposes a causal, mechanical model; the retinal image is a pattern of stimulation, and it is this stimulation that performs a vital causal role in giving rise to visual experience. The details of his positive account lie outside our present con-cerns.[19] The important point is that Descartes gives up the idea that the retinal image is perceived or experienced as a picture, and so, for him, in contrast with Kepler and Leonardo, the problem of the retinal image ceases to be a problem. For once we give up the idea that the retinal image plays a role in vision *as a picture* (i.e., as a visible depiction of something else), we lose any reason for thinking that the orientation of the retinal image is even relevant to the perceived spatial orientation of what we see. When it is viewed merely as an element in the causal process by which the visual experience is produced, there is simply no sense to the idea that the reti-nal image is even upside down. Upside down relative to what?

A similar point can be made about the problem of cyclopean vision. The existence of two retinal images only creates a problem for a unified visual experience if we suppose that we see by, as it were, perceiving the two interior pictures. Once we realize that qua pictures, the two retinal pictures are not necessary for vision, we can appreciate that there is no need to compensate for or somehow explain away the fact that there are two of them. There is no more reason to think that two retinal images should give rise to double images than there is to think that two hands should give rise to double images. Descartes writes (referring to letters in figure 2.5):

So that you must not be surprised that the objects can be seen in their true position, even though the picture they imprint upon the eye is inverted: for this is just like our blind man's being able to sense the object *B*, which is to his right, by means of his left hand, and the object *D*, which is to his left, by means of his right hand at one and the same time. And just as this blind man does not judge that a body is dou-ble, although he touches it with two hands, so likewise when both our eyes are dis-posed in the manner which is required in order to carry our attention toward one and the same location, they need only cause us to see a single object there, even though a picture of it is formed in each of our eyes. ([1637] 1965, 105)

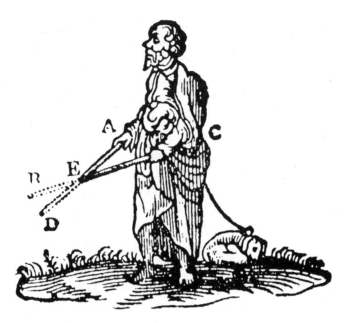

Figure 2.5
Descartes' ([1637] 1902) representation of binocular vision on the analogy of a blind
man with two sticks, from Wade 1998, 249.

Descartes' basic insight is that we cannot explain the ability to see by
positing mental pictures. If the retinal image plays a causal role in vision—
something to be established empirically—its performance of this role
cannot be due to its *pictorial* qualities.[20]

No contemporary theorist believes that we see by seeing internal pictures. Nevertheless, what I have called *the fundamental problem for visual
theory*—namely, the problem of explaining how we see what we do given
the imperfections of the retinal image—has basically the same shape as
these antique puzzles.

Consider filling in at the blind spot again. We noted above that it is
commonplace to infer the existence of a filling-in process from the fact
that we do not notice a gap in the visual field. This filling-in reasoning
is analogous to the inference to the existence of a process whereby
the retinal image is reinverted, from the fact that we experience the
visual world right-side up, or to the existence of a process of integration of the two retinal images, from the bare fact that we do not experience two visual fields. That is to say, the quick inference to the

existence of a process of filling in is fallacious; it commits the homunculus fallacy.

Dennett (1991) has insisted that we are *not* entitled to infer that there is
neural filling-in of an internal representation from the fact that we notice
no gap in the visual field (that the line appears unbroken). For this neglects
the possibility that the brain may simply *ignore* the absence of information
corresponding to the blind spot. If the brain ignores the absence of such
information—and so produces no internal representation of the absence of
the information—then there is literally nothing for the brain to fill in.
Perhaps, Dennett proposes, when you examine a wall of a uniform color,
the brain does not produce a representation that is spatially isomorphic to
the whole wall. Perhaps it simply records the fact that (or the guess that)
the wall is, say, all red, ignoring the fact that it receives no information
about the color of the wall in the region corresponding to the blind spot.
This would produce the same effect as a filling-in process—we would experience no gap in the visual field—but without the existence of a process of
filling in.

Of course this may not be what happens. To find out whether there is
filling in, we must engage in empirical study of the brain basis of consciousness (Pessoa, Thompson, and Noë 1998). But Dennett is right that,
in the absence of direct evidence of a process of filling in, we are not entitled to infer that there is any such process. It is striking that many visual
scientists—for example, Palmer as cited earlier—seem to think that to
establish the reality of filling in it is sufficient merely to observe that
we experience the visual field as gap-free, or the line as unbroken. To prove
the existence of filling in, direct evidence of the occurrence of a neural
process of filling in is needed. To assume filling in occurs in the absence of
this evidence is to commit the homunculus fallacy.[21]

Proposals to explain visual stability despite eye movement are also guilty
of committing the homunculus fallacy. Most proposals to explain visual
stability share the following assumption (as noticed by Bridgeman, Van der
Heijden, and Velichkovsky 1994): A saccadic eye movement produces a
change in the location within the brain of the brain's representation of an
object. Given this, it is natural for theorists to posit a special mechanism
of compensation to eliminate such changes in position to guarantee stability. Bridgeman, Van der Heijden, and Velichkovsky (1994) question this
move. The representation of an object's position in the world should not

be confused with the position (within the brain) of that representation. The position in a topographically organized brain map need not be the code for object position in the environment. Analogously, movement in the world need not be represented by "movement" in such maps. As Bridgeman and colleagues put it: "The idea that there is a movement perception problem when the eyes saccade arises from thinking about what happens during a saccade, and from confusing the position of representing an object in the brain with the position of the object that is represented in the world" (Bridgeman, van der Heijden, and Velichkovsky 1994, 225). Once this problematic pattern of reasoning is noticed, however, we can appreciate that there is no better reason to suppose that retinotopic movement represents real movement than there would be to suppose that the orientation of the retinal image encodes the orientation of objects in the environment, or that the number of retinal images (two) encodes the number of objects perceived. The upshot of this line of thought is that it was a mistake to believe that there *had to be* an active mechanism to compensate for retinal displacement. Once this is realized, other kinds of account can be sought.[22]

Dennett has claimed that talk of filling-in in cognitive science is a dead giveaway of vestigial "Cartesian materialism." What he has in mind is that talk of filling in seems to rely on the idea that there is a place in the brain— the Cartesian theater—where consciousness happens. The idea can be explained with reference to filling in at the blind spot again. If the brain has already determined that, say, the bar is unbroken, then for whose benefit does it perform the act of filling in? The assumption would seem to be implicit that the now filled-in content must be presented to consciousness in the Cartesian theater in order for us to have the experience as of an unbroken line.

The purpose of this section has been to reveal the extent to which our thinking about perception, like that of Leonardo and Kepler, is tied to a problematic conception of the need for pictures in the head, what theorists today might describe as internal neural structures that are spatially or topographically isomorphic to that which they represent. This conception is strictly independent of the snapshot conception. Nevertheless, it may be that if we were to give up the snapshot conception, we would find it easier to find our way clear to giving up the need for pictures in the head to underwrite our experiences.

2.3   Is Visual Experience Machian?

Let us now ask, is it really the case that our experience represents the world in sharp focus, uniform detail, and brilliant color, from the center out to the periphery of the visual field, as Mach's picture would have it? If it isn't, then vision science has been barking up the wrong tree when it seeks to explain how, on the basis of the relatively information-poor patterns of light striking the retina, we are able to enjoy colorful, detailed, high-resolution, picture-like visual experiences.

It's pretty easy to demonstrate that the snapshot conception is wrongheaded. Fix your gaze on a point straight ahead. Have a friend wave a brightly colored piece of paper off to the side. You'll immediately notice that something is moving in the periphery of your visual field, but you won't be able to tell what color it is. Ask your friend to move the paper closer to the center of the visual field. You won't be sure what color the paper is until it has been moved to within twenty to thirty degrees from the center.[23] This proves that we don't experience the periphery of our visual field in anything like the clarity, detail, or focus with which we can take in what we are directly looking at. It's tempting to say that outside that central region, we don't actually perceive colors!

Or consider the page you are now reading. Stare at a word or phrase. Without moving your eyes, how many other words can you distinctly make out? If you attend carefully, you'll notice that you can make out *very few* of the other words, even directly above or below the fixated word. There's a substantial experimental literature on reading and eye movements. In one well-known study, an eye-tracking device is driven by a computer in such a way as to change the stimulus *as the eye moves*. Readers have the experience of reading a normal page of text when in fact they are experiencing a "moving window of text" as illustrated here (taken from Grimes 1996, 94; note that the underlined letter indicates the fixation point):

XXXX XXX XXXX th̲undered XXXX XXX XXX XX X XXX

XXXX XXX XXXX XXXXXXXed in̲to the sky XX X XXX

Experiments such as this one have led some thinkers (e.g., O'Regan [1992] and Blackmore et al. [1995]) to propose that the impression we have of the presence and richness of the visual world is an illusion.[24] We have the impression that the world is represented in full detail in consciousness because, wherever we look, we encounter detail. All the detail is present, but it is only present *virtually*, for example, in the way that a web site's content is present on your desktop (Minsky 1985; Dennett 1991; O'Regan 1992; Rensink 2000). It is *as if* all the content at the remote server is *present* on your local machine, even though it isn't really. The thought was first articulated by Minsky, who wrote: "We have the sense of actuality when every question asked of our visual systems is answered so swiftly that it seems as though those answers were already there" (1985, 257).

The idea that visual awareness of detail is a kind of *virtual awareness* is consequential. (It plays an important role in chapters 4 and 7 of this book.) It is tantamount to the rejection of the orthodoxy that vision is the process whereby a rich internal representation of experienced detail is built up. If experiences are not Machian—as these considerations would seem to demonstrate—then efforts to explain how the brain can give rise to the sort of detailed internal representations needed to subserve such experiences are misdirected. To experience detail virtually, you don't *need* to have all the detail in your head. All you need is quick and easy access to the relevant detail when you need it. Just as you don't need to download, say, the entire *New York Times* to be able to read it on your desktop, so you don't need to construct a representation of all the detail of the scene in front of you to have a sense of its detailed presence.

Virtual representation has both advantages and disadvantages. In the Internet case, the disadvantages are clear: You are beholden to the network; if it goes down, you've got none of the resources at hand. But the advantages are also clear: given that you *are* networked, it's cheaper and simpler to make use of what is already available on the remote site. There's no need to go through the expense of reduplicating that information on one's own hard drive. Moreover, you can let the server managers bear the costs of updating content. Whenever you log on to the web site, you can read the latest news.

The advantages of virtual representation in vision are comparable. There's no need to build up a detailed internal model of the world. The world is right there and can serve as "its own best model" (Brooks 1991). O'Regan (1992) makes the same point when he proposes that the world can serve as an "outside memory"; there's no need to *re*-present the world on one's own internal memory drive. Off-loading internal processing onto the world simplifies our cognitive lives and makes good engineering and evolutionary sense.[25]

But there are disadvantages too. Just as in the Internet case we are beholden to the network, so in this case we are beholden to our continued access to the visual world, an access that depends on the detailed nature of our bodies and the way we are environmentally situated. We *don't* have the detailed world in consciousness all at once. Our contact with that world is just that much more tenuous. This tenuousness is illustrated by change blindness, a psychological phenomenon discovered in the course of trying to establish that vision does not depend on internal representations.

To set the stage, suppose I say to you as you begin to eat your lunch: "Hey? Isn't that Mick Jagger over there?" You turn around to look. When you do, I snatch one of your french fries. When you turn back, you're none the wiser. You don't remember the exact number or layout of fries on your plate, and you weren't paying attention when the fry was snatched.

It's not news to be told in this way that we are *difference blind*, as Dretske (2004) has put it. We're blind to the difference between, for example, the look of the plate of fries before and after the theft. A standard children's puzzle is to study two pictures to see if you can discover the difference between them. The settled upshot of change blindness research conducted by O'Regan, Rensink, Simons and Levin, and others,[26] is that this sort of failure to notice change in the french fries case is a pervasive feature of our visual lives. We are not merely difference blind, we are frequently *change* blind, that is, blind to changes even when they occur directly in front of us in full view.

Usually, when changes occur before us, we notice them, because our attention is grabbed by the flickers of movement associated with the change (as we would immediately notice the moving piece of colored paper in the periphery of our visual field). This is explained by properties of cells in the parafoveal region of the retina. But if we are prevented from noticing the flicker of movement when the change occurs—say, because at the same time flickers occur elsewhere—we may fail to notice the change (O'Regan, Rensink, and Clark 1996, 1999). We will frequently fail to notice changes even when the changes are fully open to view. Even when we are looking right at the change when it occurs, something we can test with eye trackers, we may fail to see the change (O'Regan et al. 2000). In one noteworthy recent demonstration, carried out by Kevin O'Regan, you are shown a photograph of a Paris street scene. Over the seconds that you look at the picture, the color of a car prominently displayed in the foreground changes from red to blue. Perceivers overwhelmingly fail to notice this change in color, even though the change is dramatic and occurs over a short period of time. When the color change is pointed out, perceivers laugh aloud and express astonishment that they could have failed to miss the change.

It is sometimes said that change blindness shows that there are no detailed internal representations. It does not show this. Change blindness is compatible with the existence of detailed internally stored information about what is present to vision. Indeed, a number of recent studies demonstrate that subjects, when questioned appropriately, reveal a good deal of information about features in a scene whose variation they had failed to notice. For example, in one study a person is asked for directions by a young woman in athletic dress holding a basketball; subjects tend not to notice that at some moment when there is a distraction, the basketball is replaced with a volleyball. Although subjects failed to notice the switch, they were more likely, when questioned later, to give accurate "guesses" about, say, whether when first approached the woman was holding one kind of ball rather than another.[27]

Change blindness is evidence, then, that the representations needed to subserve vision *could* be virtual. Change blindness suggests that we don't make use of detailed internal models of the scene (even if it doesn't show that there are no detailed internal representations). In normal perception it seems that we don't have online access to detailed internal representations of the scene.

Change blindness has other important implications. One of these is that vision is, to some substantial degree, attention-dependent (e.g., Rensink, O'Regan, and Clark 1997). If a change takes place when attention is directed elsewhere, the change will tend to go unnoticed. In general, you only see that to which you attend. If something occurs outside the scope of attention, even if it's perfectly visible (i.e., unobstructed, central, large), you won't see it. A striking example comes from the literature on the related phenomenon of inattentional blindness.[28] In a now famous study, perceivers are asked to watch a videotape of a basketball game and to count the number of times one team takes possession of the ball (Neisser 1976; Simons and Chabris 1999). During the film clip (see figure 2.6), which lasts a few minutes, a person in a gorilla suit strolls onto the center of the field of play, turns and faces the audience, and does a little jig. The gorilla then slowly walks off the court. The remarkable fact is that perceivers (including this author) *do not* notice the gorilla.

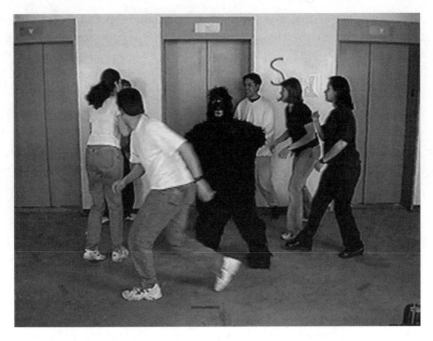

Figure 2.6
Viewers attending to the play may fail to notice the gorilla (Simons and Chabris 1999). This is an example of inattentional blindness.

A second apparent implication of the change blindness/inattentional blindness work is more philosophical. It has been hinted at already. Change blindness and inattentional blindness would seem to show that we are victims of an illusion about the character of our own experience. It seems to us that we enjoy a visual impression of the environment in sharp focus and detail. But we do not! The experience of detail is an illusion. Traditional philosophical skepticism about perception questions whether we can know, on the basis of experience, that things are the way we experience them as being. Change blindness suggests a new sort of skepticism about experience. This new skepticism calls into question whether we even really know how things perceptually seem to us. Perceptual consciousness, according to this new skepticism, is a kind of false consciousness. In this vein, O'Regan writes: "despite the poor quality of the visual apparatus, we have the subjective impression of great richness and 'presence' of the visual world. But this richness and presence are actually an illusion" (1992, 484).[29]

A similar thought is expressed by Susan Blackmore and her colleagues, who write: "We believe that we see a complete, dynamic picture of a stable, uniformly detailed, and colourful world," but "[o]ur stable visual world may be constructed out of a brief retinal image and a very sketchy, higher-level representation along with a pop-out mechanism to redirect attention. The richness of our visual world is, to this extent, an illusion" (Blackmore et al. 1995, 1075).

The thinker who has done most to articulate the new skepticism and give it punch is Daniel Dennett (and he did so *before* the discovery of change blindness; indeed, he actually predicted change blindness; see Dennett 1991, 467–468).[30] Edelman had written, "One of the most striking things about consciousness is its continuity" (1989, 119). Dennett writes in response: "This is utterly wrong. One of the most striking features about consciousness is its discontinuity—as revealed in the blind spot, and saccadic gaps, to take the simplest examples. The discontinuity of consciousness is striking because of the *apparent* continuity of consciousness" (1991, 356).

This remark makes very clear that the worry is about the nature of experience or consciousness itself. Dennett's claim is that we are misled as to the true nature of consciousness. Consciousness is *really* discontinuous. It *appears to us* to be continuous. A paradoxical way to put the point would be: It turns out that we are mistaken in our assessment of how things seem to us be. This is a skeptical proposal more radical than anything Descartes would have found intelligible!

We can get a handle on Dennett's skeptical reasoning in connection with his discussion of filling in at the blind spot. As noted earlier, Dennett thinks talk of filling in reveals a bad philosophical theory of consciousness. Arguments for filling in are frequently not grounded on evidence of a process of neural filling in but are rather driven by philosophical dogma about what *must happen* to give rise to experience as we know it. If, as a matter of empirical fact, there is no filling in, then (given Dennett's background assumptions) it follows that we are deluded as to the character of our visual experience. It seems as if there's no gap in visual experience, even when one fixates on a uniformly colored surface with one eye. But given that the brain doesn't fill in, it follows that there *is* a gap in our experience of the wall, a gap we simply fail to recognize. This is an example of the *apparent continuity* of what is in fact a genuinely discontinuous phenomenon. We're the victims of an illusion of consciousness.

Dennett offers a second example, the visual experience of wallpaper with a repeating pattern. Suppose you are looking at wallpaper that is covered with a repeating photographic image of Marilyn Monroe's face. When you enter the room, it looks to you as if you see that the wall is covered with Marilyns. But you certainly don't foveate each of them in series; owing to the limitations of foveal and parafoveal vision, you don't take them *all* in all at once. You can't make out the Marilyns in the periphery of your visual field in sufficient detail. One way to explain our impression of all the Marilyns—this would be the filling-in proposal—is that the brain builds up (i.e., *fills in*) a representation of each of the Marilyns, as it were, across an internal screen. An alternative—the anti-filling-in proposal Dennett favors—is that the brain detects a few Marilyns and then "jumps to the conclusion" that the rest are Marilyns too. If this is in fact what happens, then the brain does not produce a representation sufficient to give rise to the experience of hundreds of Marilyns. Your impression that you see hundreds of them is an illusion! Note that there's no perceptual illusion; you correctly judge that there are hundreds of Marilyns. The illusion is an illusion of consciousness: You don't really experience them all, even though you think you do. As philosophers would say, you don't really have an experience *as of* hundreds of Marilyns. Dennett writes: "Having identified a single Marilyn, and having received no information to the effect that the other blobs are not Marilyns, it [the brain] jumps to the conclusion that the rest are Marilyns, and labels the whole region 'more Marilyns' without any further rendering of Marilyns at all. Of course it does not seem that way to you. It seems to you as if you are actually seeing hundreds of identical Marilyns" (1991, 335).

It seems to you as if you are actually experiencing hundreds of Marilyns when, in fact, you are not. The absence of an internal representation of all the Marilyns means that you lack the internal substrate necessary for the having of that experience. Your perceptual experience of the Marilyns is a confabulation.

2.4   Is the Visual World a Grand Illusion?

Are we radically misguided as to the character of our own conscious experience, as Dennett and others have argued? Do the arguments of the new skeptic, based on considerations about change blindness and the blind spot, succeed? I think not.[31]

Let's consider the case of the blind spot first. It is certainly right that you don't notice a gap in the visual field corresponding to the blind spot, even under monocular viewing conditions. In general, if you shut one eye and stare at the wall with the other, you have a visual experience as of a gap-free expanse of the wall. That is, it looks to you as if there is an unbroken expanse of wall. But this is not to say that it seems to you as if, as it were in a single fixation, you experience *the whole of the wall's surface.* If you reflect on what it is like for you to look at the wall, you will notice that it seems to you as if the whole wall is there, at once, but not as if every part of the wall's surface is represented in your consciousness at once. Rather, you experience the wall as present, and you experience yourself as having access to the wall, by looking here, or there, by attending here, or there. It is no part of ordinary phenomenology that we experience the whole wall, every bit of it, in consciousness, all at once.[32]

We can make the same sort of point about the Marilyn Monroe wallpaper example. "It seems to you as if you are actually seeing hundreds of identical Marilyns" (Dennett 1991). This is right, on one construal, but it's wrong on another. It's wrong if it is meant to suggest that it seems to you, now, while you are attentively fixing your gaze at a point on the wall, that you have *all* the Marilyns in clear focus. When you fixate on a point on the wall, you can't see all the Marilyns, nor does it seem to you as if you can. You can see clearly what is right there at the center of your focus (the part of the wall corresponding to your foveal region). But the many Marilyns that are outside your focus do not seem to you to be present in sharp focus and high-resolution detail. True, they seem to be present, but not in the way that Mach's picture would suggest they are present. But it is only this Machian seeing of all the Marilyns—having all the Marilyns in clear view at once—that is upset by the consideration that there is no detailed internal representation of all the Marilyns. Dennett's claim—"It seems to you as if you are actually seeing hundreds of identical Marilyns"—is right only if we take it to mean, roughly, that one takes oneself, on the basis of vision, to have a sense of the presence of the wall as covered with Marilyns.

The crux is this: The skeptical reasoning relies on a bad inference from the character of a single visual fixation to the character of seeing itself. From the fact that, when I stare at a point on the wall, I can't see colors in the periphery, it doesn't follow that there are no colors in the periphery of the visual field. For my visual field—my visual world—is not the field available to the fixed gaze. The visual field, rather, is made available by *looking around*. We look here, then there, and in this way we gain access to the world and our experience acquires that world as content. It is no part of our phenomenological commitments that we take ourselves to have all that detail at hand *in a single fixation*.

The skeptical argument seems to turn on attributing to us, as lay perceivers, something very much like Mach's snapshot conception of experience. According to this conception, visual experiences are like snapshots that represent the scene in high-resolution focus and sharp detail. The skeptic then points out, convincingly, that our experience is not like a snapshot—there's a blind spot, bad parafoveal vision, and so forth—and he or she concludes that we are victims of an illusion about the character of our own consciousness.

But the mistake in question—the snapshot conception of experience, Mach's picture—is not one to which lay perceivers themselves are committed. Perhaps it is an idea about perception that psychologists or philosophers find natural. Perhaps it is a way of describing experience that many ordinary perceivers would be inclined to assent to if they were asked appropriately leading questions. But this is compatible with its being the case that we do not really take our experience to be this way.

Exactly similar remarks can be made about change blindness. It just is not the case that we, normal perceivers, "believe we see a complete, dynamic picture of a stable, uniformly detailed and colorful world," as Blackmore and her colleagues suggested (see the earlier quotation).[33] Of course it *does* seem to us as if we have perceptual access to a world that is richly detailed, complete, and gap-free. And indeed we do! We take ourselves to be confronted with and embedded in a high-resolution environment. We take ourselves to have access to that detail, not all at once, but thanks to movements of our eyes and head and shifts of attention.[34]

Consider a question posed by Rensink: "Why do we feel that somewhere in our brain is a complete, coherent representation of the entire scene?" (2000, 28). But this question rests on a false presupposition. It does *not* seem to us as if somewhere in our brain there is a complete, coherent representation of the scene. Perceptual experience is directed to the world, not to the brain.

If I am right that perceivers are not committed to the idea that they have detailed pictures in the head when they see (the snapshot conception), then how can we explain the fact that perceivers are surprised by the results of change blindness? Does not the surprise itself register our commitment to the problematic, snapshot conception of experience? This objection has been raised by Dennett:

> why do normal perceivers express such surprise when their attention is drawn to [the relevant facts about their perceptual limitations]. Surprise is a wonderful dependent variable, and should be used more often in experiments; it is easy to measure and is a telling betrayal of the subject's *having expected something else*. These expectations are, indeed, an overshooting of the proper expectations of a normally embedded perceiver-agent; people shouldn't have these expectations, but they do. People are shocked, incredulous, dismayed; they often laugh and shriek when I demonstrate the effects to them for the first time. These behavioral responses are themselves data in good standing, and in need of an explanation. (2001, 982; see also 2002)

This is an important objection, but one that is easy to counter. The astonishment people experience when confronted with the facts of change blindness and inattentional blindness does indeed demonstrate that their beliefs are upset by these demonstrations.[35] But one need not attribute to them (to us) a commitment to the snapshot conception. The surprise is explained simply by supposing that we tend to think we are better at noticing changes than we in fact are, or that we are much less vulnerable to the effects of distracted attention than we in fact are. This is a plausible explanation of the surprise we feel when confronted with the results, and one that does not foist on us the ideology of the snapshot conception.

Surprise requires explanation, but so does the lack of surprise. Notice that we are *not* surprised or in any way taken aback by our need, in the course of daily living, to move eyes and head to get better glimpses of what is around us. We peer, squint, lean forward, adjust lighting, put on glasses, and we do so automatically. The fact that we are not surprised by our lack of immediate possession of detailed information about the environment shows that we don't take ourselves to have all that information in consciousness all at once. If we were committed to the snapshot conception, wouldn't we be surprised by the need to redirect our attention continuously to the environment to inform ourselves about what is there?

Finally, it is worth noting that artists, magicians, stage designers, and cinematographers—people who live by the maxim that the hand is quicker than the eye—would not be surprised by the change blindness results. Why should they be? Our perceptual access to the world is robust, but fallible and vulnerable. How could one really think otherwise? An artist friend of mine, working on a portrait series, asked me to sit for him. I was struck by the frenzy of his looking-activity. The rendering proceeded by means of an uninterrupted pattern of looking back and forth from me to the canvas. The detail wasn't in his memory, or in his internal representations. It was to be found in his subject (in me).

Let us summarize what we have found so far. First, the new skepticism is right about some things. For example, it is right that experience does not conform to the snapshot conception. And so it is right that vision science should not concern itself with how the brain produces experiences thought of like that. But the new skepticism seems to rest on a substantially false characterization of what perceptual experience actually seems to us—that is, to lay perceivers—to be like. In particular, it attributes to us something like the snapshot conception. The skepticism can be resisted if we recognize that we are not committed to the snapshot conception. We don't take ourselves to experience all environmental detail in consciousness all at once. Rather, we take ourselves to be situated in an environment, to have access to environmental detail as needed by turns of the eyes and head and by repositioning of the body.

2.5   The Problem of Perceptual Presence

We are not done yet. We must not be too quick to dismiss the hypothesis that the visual world is a grand illusion. One of the results of change blindness is that we only see, we only experience, that to which we attend. But surely it is a basic fact of our phenomenology that we enjoy a perceptual awareness of at least some unattended features of the scene. So, for example, I may look at you, attending only to you. But I also have a sense of the presence of the wall behind you in the background, of its color, of its distance from you. It certainly seems this way. If we are not to fall back into the grip of the new skepticism, we must explain how it is we can enjoy perceptual experience of unattended features of a scene. Let us call this the problem of perceptual presence.

More generally, we can ask: In what does our sense of the presence of the detailed environment consist, if not in the fact that we see it? How can it seem to us as if the world is present to us visually in all its detail without its seeming to us as if we *see* all that detail?

The problem of perceptual presence forces us to confront the grand illusion puzzle again. But this version of the puzzle is stronger, for it does not rely on the misattribution to us of the phenomenologically inadequate snapshot conception of experience. All that it requires is that we acknowledge that we are perceptually aware, sometimes, of unattended detail. And who could deny that?

To begin to see our way clear to a solution of the problem of perceptual presence, consider, as an example, a perceptual experience such as that you might enjoy if you were to hold a bottle in your hands with eyes closed.[36] You have a sense of the presence of a whole bottle, even though you only make contact with the bottle at a few isolated points. Can we explain how your experience in this way outstrips what is actually given, or must we concede that your sense of the bottle as a whole is a kind of confabulation?

Or consider a different case: A cat sits motionless on the far side of a picket fence. You have a sense of the presence of a cat even though, strictly speaking, you only see those parts of the cat that show through the fence. How is it that we can in this way enjoy a perceptual experience as of the whole cat?

These are instances of the problem of perceptual presence. We have a sense of the presence of that which, strictly speaking, we do not perceive.

One way we might try to explain this phenomenon is by observing that to experience the cat or the bottle as voluminous wholes requires that you draw on your knowledge of what bottles are, or what cats are. You bring to bear your conceptual skills. This is doubtless right. To experience the cat *as* a cat, or *as* a whole, is to experience what you see as falling under concepts. But this can't be the whole story. For what we want is an account not of our *thought* or *judgment* or *belief* that, say, there is a whole bottle there, or a whole cat there. What we want is an account of our *perceptual sense* of their presence.

Crucially—and this is a phenomenological point—the cat and the bottle seem present as wholes, *perceptually*. The strictly unseen environmental detail seems perceptually present even though we do not see it all at once. We do not merely *think* that these features are present. Indeed, this sense of perceptual presence does not depend on the availability of the corresponding belief.

This last point is illustrated by a consideration of figure 2.7, an illustration of Kanizsa's. We naturally perceive this figure as the depiction of a triangle partially occluding three disks. We don't merely *think* the presence of the occluded bits: After all, they are, evidently, *not* present, but blocked from view (or rather, not drawn); it *looks* as if they are blocked from view. We experience the presence of the occluded bits even as we experience, plainly, their absence. They are present *as absent*.[37] Our sense of the perceptual presence of the disks is not significantly altered by the explicit recognition that there are not really occluded bits present.

This phenomenon is an example of what psychologists call *amodal perception*. We experience the occluded portions of the disks in the Kanizsa figure as *amodally* present in perception. They are *perceptually* present without being actually perceived. This phenomenon—perceptual presence, amodal seeing—is very widespread in perception. As examples we can count the cases we've already mentioned—the experience of the environment as detailed despite the fact that we don't actually attend to or

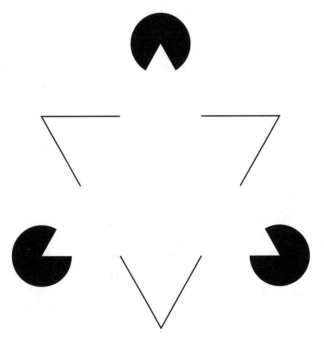

Figure 2.7
Kanisza triangle: The contours of the upper triangle are illusory.

notice all the detail, the experience of the cat behind the fence as a whole, the experience of the bottle as whole despite the fact that we only touch parts of it—but there are many other instances of the phenomenon, for example, the visual experience of voluminousness, as, for example, when you experience a tomato as three-dimensional and round, even though you only see its facing side, or the experience of a chair as whole and intact, even though it is partially blocked from view by the table. Another example is color constancy; we experience the wall as a uniform shade despite the fact that it is visibly different with respect to color in different places, depending on illumination. (I discuss this further in chapter 4.)

To understand the phenomenon of perceptual presence, then, is not only to get clear about the grand illusion problem posed by the new skepticism, it is also to understand a class of central perceptual phenomena (phenomena that are not typically grouped together).

Traditional orthodoxy addresses the problem of perceptual presence by supposing that we build up an internal model corresponding to, say, experienced detail. This sort of approach faces obstacles that we have already considered. For example, work on change blindness calls into question whether in perception we make use of such detailed internal models.

But there are more fundamental reasons to question the orthodox strategy. Why should the brain go to the trouble of producing a model of the bottle when the bottle is right there to serve as a repository of information about itself? All the information about the bottle you need is available to you in the world—you need only move your hands to gather it. And so for the cat. Why should the brain need to represent the cat in all its detail, when all the information you need is available when you need it by eye and head movements (Dreyfus [1972] 1992; Minsky 1985; Brooks 1991; O'Regan 1992; Clark 1997)?

I would like to suggest that the popularity of the orthodox strategy stems from the implicit assumption of the snapshot conception of experience. Many thinkers implicitly assume that when we see, we represent the whole scene in consciousness all at once. I have urged us to admit that this assumption is wrongheaded, that it amounts to a distorting misdescription of our phenomenology. It does not seem to me as if every part of the cat is visible to me now, even though it does seem to me, now, as if I perceive a whole cat and as if the unperceived parts of the cat's body are present. After all, I can *see* that the cat is partly hidden behind the fence! This is just the thing with amodal perception: One experiences the presence of that which one perceives to be *out of view*.

This phenomenological admonishment is the key, I think, to the whole problem. If we get clearer about the phenomenology in the way I am suggesting, then we can see that our sense of the perceptual presence of the cat as a whole now does not require us to be committed to the idea that we represent the whole cat in consciousness at once. What it requires, rather, is that we take ourselves to have *access*, now, to the whole cat. The cat, the tomato, the bottle, the detailed scene, all are present perceptually in the sense that they are perceptually accessible to us. They are present to perception as accessible. They are, in this sense, *virtually* present.

The ground of this accessibility is our possession of sensorimotor skills (O'Regan and Noë 2001a,b). In particular, the basis of perceptual presence is to be found in those skills whose possession is constitutive, in the ways I have been proposing, of sensory perception. My relation to the cat behind the fence is mediated by such facts as that, when I blink, I lose sight of it altogether, but when I move a few inches to the right, a part of its side that was previously hidden comes into view. My sense of the perceptual presence, now, of that which is now hidden behind a slat in the fence, consists in my expectation that by moving my body I can produce the right sort of "new cat" stimulation.

In this way, we can explain our sense of the perceptual presence of, say, the whole tomato. Our perceptual sense of the tomato's wholeness—of its volume and backside, and so forth—consists in our implicit understanding (our expectation) that movements of our body to the left or right, say, will bring further bits of the tomato into view. Our relation to the unseen bits of the tomato is mediated by patterns of sensorimotor contingency. Similar points can be made across the board for occlusion phenomena.

In general, our sense of the perceptual presence of the detailed world does not consist in our representation of all the detail in consciousness now. Rather, it consists in our access now to all of the detail, and to our knowledge that we have this access. This knowledge takes the form of our comfortable mastery of the rules of sensorimotor dependence that mediate our relation to the cat and the bottle. My sense of the presence of the whole cat behind the fence consists precisely in my knowledge, my implicit understanding, that by a movement of the eye or the head or the body, I can bring bits of the cat into view that are now hidden. This is one of the central claims of the enactive or sensorimotor approach to perception (O'Regan and Noë 2001a,b).

You also have a sense of the presence of the room next door, for example. But your sense of its presence is not a sense of its *perceptual* presence. It doesn't seem to you now, for example, as if you *see* the space on the other side of the wall. This is explained by the fact that your relation to the room next door is not mediated by the kinds of patterns of sensori- motor dependence in the way that your relation to the tomato and the cat and the detailed environment is (O'Regan and Noë 2001a). For example, you can jump up and down, turn around, turn the lights on and off, blink, and so on, and it makes no difference whatsoever to your sense of the presence of the room next door.

Can this be right? One problem is that even though you obviously do not visually experience the room next door, your relation to that room is no less mediated by patterns of sensorimotor dependence than is your rela- tion to the back of the tomato, or to the cat behind the picket fence. Certainly, movements of your body in respect of the room next door are such as to be able to bring it into view. You just have to walk over there. The theory would seem, then, to have the unintended consequence that we *do* see the room next door. In this sense the theory is too strong. A sec- ond problem runs the other way; I have argued that you do have a sense of the perceptual presence of the occluded portions of the tomato, even though you don't see them. Is the theory strong enough to explain this? In what sense is your relation to the hidden portion of the tomato *visual*? You wouldn't see an ant crawling across it.

The theory does have the resources to reply to these objections. To do so, we need to differentiate two different kinds of sensorimotor relation. Our sensory relation to the world varies along two dimensions. The relation is *movement*-dependent when the slightest movements of the body modulate sensory stimulation. But when you see an object, your relation to it is also *object*-dependent; that is, movements *of the object* produce sensory change. In general, when you see x, your relation to it is both movement- and object-dependent. (The object dependence of sensory stimulation, we have noticed, plays an important role in explaining the ability to perceive change.) To perceive an object, in general, is to deploy sensorimotor skills of both sorts; perceivers are familiar with not only the sensory effects of movement, but also the sensory effects produced by environmental changes.

The bearing of this distinction on the first problem is as follows: Your relation to the room next door is not perceptual, even though it is movement-dependent, because the relation is not object-dependent. Movements or changes in the room next door will not provoke (visual) sensory change. In addition, although your relation to the room next door is movement-dependent, it is less movement-dependent than your relation to the tomato in front of you. Blinking affects your relation to the tomato in front of you, but not to the room next door.

As for the second problem—that we don't really see the hidden parts of the tomato—consider that, not only is it the case that your relation to the tomato is highly movement-dependent, it is also object-dependent: If the far side of the tomato were to move, this would be likely to attract your attention. True, you don't see an ant crawling across it. But this is exactly the consequence one wants: After all, in no sense is the ant perceptually present.[38]

In general, these considerations reveal that the difference between the sense of the perceptual presence of something strictly unseen (the back of the tomato) and the sense of the (nonperceptual) presence of an unseen item (the room next door) are matters of degree.

2.6   Overintellectualizing the Mind: A Reply to Dreyfus

The solution to the problem of perceptual presence turns on admitting that perception is constituted not only by the perceiver's mastery of patterns of sensorimotor dependence, but by the fact that the perceiver *knows* that his or her relation to the environment is mediated by such knowledge. The need for this further knowledge is clear: How can you experience a strictly unseen bit of an occluded surface as perceptually present? Your sense of its presence cannot be explained simply by reference to the fact that you receive stimulation from it. Because, when it is occluded, you do not. Nor is your perceptual sense of the presence of the occluded surface explained by the mere fact that your relation to that surface is mediated by patterns of sensorimotor dependence. All that can explain your sense now of the perceptual presence of what is really unperceived is your grasp, now, that your relation to the occluded surface is mediated by the relevant sensorimotor contingencies. It is this knowledge that makes the potential effects of your movement relevant to what you now experience.

Hubert Dreyfus (personal communication), developing a Heideggerian position, has questioned whether the enactive approach, as I have developed it here, threatens to overintellectualize the mind by supposing that the ground of our sensorimotor skill is intellectual knowledge about the character of one's relation to the environment. Drawing on ideas of Heidegger, he urges that we think of our perceptual engagement with the world as a form of "skillful coping" that need not depend on any *knowledge* about the character of one's relation to the world.

I am sypathetic to this line of criticism, but I think that the enactive approach has the resources to defend itself. The facts are these: Perceivers continuously move about and modify their relation to the environment. They do this in order to get better vantage points and to bring themselves into contact with the relevant detail that is of interest. In this way they exhibit not merely skillful mastery of the ways sensory stimulation varies as they move, but also expectations about the effect of movements on their access to the environment. These latter expectations reflect the kind of knowledge to which we have found it necessary to appeal to explain perceptual presence. Perceivers have an implicit, practical understanding of the way movements produce changes in sensory stimulation. They also have an implicit practical understanding that they are coupled to the world in such a way that movements produce sensory change. It is this implicit practical understanding that forms the basis of their readiness to move about to find out how things are.[39]

2.7 Virtual Content and the Grand Illusion

The enactive approach to perception—with its emphasis on the centrality of our possession of sensorimotor skills—provides the basis for a satisfying reply to what I have been calling the new skepticism, but only provided that we adopt a more plausible phenomenology of perceptual experience. On this more plausible account, it is not the case that we take ourselves, when we see, for example, to represent the whole scene in consciousness all at once. The enactive, sensorimotor approach offers an explanation of how it can be that we enjoy an experience of worldly detail that is not represented in our brains. The detail is present—the perceptual world is present—in the sense that we have a special kind of access to the detail, an access controlled by patterns of sensorimotor dependence with which we are familiar.

We can epitomize this phenomenological insight as follows: The content of perceptual experience is *virtual*. This point goes beyond the proposal that the visual system utilizes virtual representations; the claim is that experiential content is itself virtual. According to the enactive approach, the far side of the tomato, the occluded portions of the cat, and the unseen environmental detail are present to perception virtually in the sense that we experience their presence because of our skill-based access to them. Phenomenological reflection on the character of perceptual presence suggests that the features are present *as available*, rather than as represented. The world is within reach and is present only insofar as we know (or feel) that it is.

Crucially, phenomenologically speaking, *virtual* presence is a kind of presence, not a kind of non-presence or illusory presence. I return to this idea in chapters 4 and 7.

2.8 The Blind Spot Revisited

Perceptual experience has an ineliminable *amodal* element. I experience the world as present even when the detail is hidden from view. Just as I experience the three-dimensionality of the tomato before me, so I experience the detail spread out before me. My experience of all that detail consists in my knowing that I have access to it all, and in the fact that I do in fact have this access. But this solution to the problem of perceptual presence—which is really the problem of perceptual content—depends on rethinking our perceptual phenomenology. In particular, we must clearly recognize that our experience, in whatever modality, is not Machian.

With these points in mind, let us reconsider the blind spot. We agreed with Palmer that when the break in the line (in figure 2.2) falls on the blind spot, the line comes to look unbroken. But now we need to be more attentive to the actual character of this visual phenomenon. Does it look unbroken in the *modal* sense, or in the *amodal* sense? Do you really experience an unbroken line? Do you really see its continuity, or merely fail to notice its break? I think it is clear that the completion of the line is, phenomenologically speaking, *a*modal. Run the demonstration again. Does it look to you as if you can *see* the unbroken space filled in? It does not. Rather, you simply don't see (can't see) the gap. We experience the space as filled in only in the sense that we experience the disks in the Kanizsa triangle (figure 2.7) as completed behind the occluding triangle. In the Kanizsa figure case, of course, we are dealing with an illusion. In fact, there is no disk behind the triangle. The display is a line drawing. And so, in the filling-in case, the line is in fact broken. My proposal—and here I am following Durgin, Tripathy, and Levi (1995)—is that blind-spot filling in is a species of amodal completion. The blind spot functions as an occluder or blocker. Features that fall on the blind spot are blocked from view in just the way that objects that are blocked from view by a hand (say, as when you hold up your hand and block your view of part of a table). And just as we experience the world as present behind occluders, so we experience the world as present "behind" the blind spot. We can demonstrate this by considering the effect of shutting an eye and holding up your thumb so that it blocks your view of the break in the line in figure 2.2. There is a sense in which the line looks complete again, only now the amodal character of its completion is evident. Crucially, the sense of the presence of that which is occluded by an object and that which is occluded by the blind spot can be explained in one and the same way: by our implicit understanding that by movements of the eye, or head, we can bring the hidden detail into view. We take it that our relation to the items that are now *out of view* is mediated by the very same patterns of sensorimotor dependence as are our relations to things that are in view. (In this case, however, we are dealing with nonveridical perception.)

From the standpoint of this enactive account, there is no need for a neural process of filling in to explain the percept; the experience acquires content thanks to our exercise of sensorimotor skills.

It is important to underscore an aspect of this discovery that is almost always overlooked. Psychologists dazzle their students with remarks to the effect that we experience the region as filled in. What is controversial is whether, to explain the percept, we need to suppose a neural process of filling in. The personal-level fact—that we experience a region in which there is no discontinuity—is taken as settled.[40] The controversy is thought to pertain only to the subpersonal level (i.e., to the question of which neural processes give rise to the personal-level perceptual content)?

I now want to propose that there is a sense in which it is *wrong* to say that it looks as if the line is unbroken.[41] It is wrong to say this in just the same way it would be wrong to say that we *really* see completed portions of the disk, in the Kanizsa triangle, or that we see the hidden portions of the cat behind the fence. There is all the difference in the world between seeing a cat behind a fence and seeing a cat that isn't partially obstructed by a fence. And there's all the difference in the world—phenomenologically, I mean—between seeing an unbroken line, and seeing a broken line whose break is made to fall on the blind spot. In the latter case, it *does* look like an unbroken line *but only in the sense that* the break is hidden from view, by the blind spot, and one *expects* that were one to move one's eyes to the right one would encounter no discontinuity.

Psychologists frequently *misdescribe* the illusory percepts they investigate. Consider the Kansiza figure again. Part of what makes this figure interesting is that it exhibits not only *amodal* completion, but also a type of *modal* completion. In particular, it exemplifies the phenomenon of *illusory contours*. The contours of the uppermost triangle are illusory contours that are, as psychologists say, induced by the cuts in the "pacmen" at the vertices. Now, there is no question that we see contours where, in fact, there are none. The illusion is robust. But notice that there is a striking difference between the experience of a triangle whose boundary is illusory, and one whose boundary is real (either because it is actually drawn in, or because there is a genuine luminance contrast). Compare figure 2.7 with the two images in figure 2.8. Illusory contours look like contours, but genuine contours don't look like illusory contours.

Considerations of this sort indicate that we need to be much more careful when describing illusory percepts in the terms used to describe their nonillusory counterparts. In particular, it shows that we cannot, without further ado, draw conclusions about normal perception from our analysis of illusory cases.[42] We need to pay greater attention to the phenomenology of our experiences.

2.9 The Visual Field

The proposed solution to the problem of perceptual presence is meant to show how it can be that we enjoy perceptual experiences that represent the world in detail, without supposing that visual experiences represent

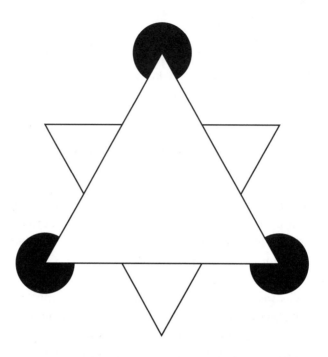

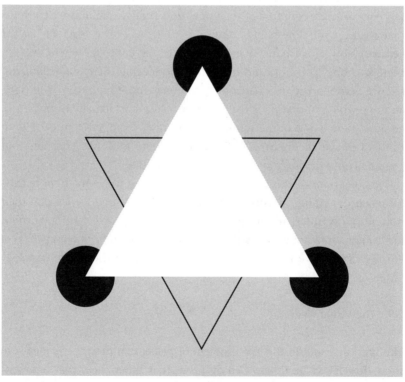

Figure 2.8
Nonillusory contours.

the way pictures do. Andreas Gursky's photograph of the interior of a Los Angeles 99 Cents Shop calls this to mind. Part of the effect of Gursky's piece is that it presents a "view" of the shop that is utterly contrived. We never *experience* so much detail, not all at once like that, as if in a picture.

There are other important aspects of experience that are nonpictorial. For example, the visual field is unbounded; there is a sense in which there is no limit to it. This can be explained on the enactive account. The unboundedness of the visual field consists in the fact that we have, and we know we have, easy access to what is now further to the right, or left, or up, or down, and so forth. The unboundedness of the field derives from the unboundedness of our sensorimotor capacities.

Or consider your experience, for example, of a gaggle of geese flying overhead. Do you experience them all? In a sense, yes. You see the gaggle. Suppose there were forty birds flying by. That's the number of birds you experienced. But you did not experience them *as forty*. Your experience would not have been any different had there been 39 birds, or 41. This is made clear in figure 2.9.

The figure on the left has 23 1s, and the figure on the right, 24. But this difference is not visible. Visual experience is not that sharply resolved. Mach's drawing distorts this characteristic indeterminacy. Wittgenstein once believed that this sort of difference showed that physical language—used to describe the world of physical things—and phenomenological language—used to describe experience—are incommensurable. A thousand-sided closed plane figure is not a circle in physical space (or in geometrical space), but in *visual space* (and visual geometry) it is. Wittgenstein thought that Mach's picture illustrated what happens when one uses a pictorial method to try to depict, not the physical, but the experiential. At best, one depicts the physical. Crucially, the vagueness in the picture (say, at the periphery) is nothing like the vagueness that characterizes the periphery of the field when we are staring straight ahead.

(a) 111111111111111111111111 (b) 1111111111111111111111111

Figure 2.9
The figure on the left has 23 1s, the figure on the right 24. Do you experience this difference?

Wittgenstein was certainly right about one thing. As we have seen, we lack skill in carefully describing what we see. We too readily describe the world we see, rather than the world *as seen*. This is sloppy, and it leads us to neglect, among other things, the differences between amodal and modal seeing, or the differences between veridical perceptual experiences and their nonveridical counterparts.

There is another sense, however, in which our failure to attend to the seeing as such can be a source of insight. The reason we don't experience things as vague, even though our visual field is indeterminate at the edges (as it were) is that, in an important sense, we don't experience our visual fields. We experience the world. The limitations of Mach's picture reveal this: It attempts to depict the visual field but ends up depicting the room as seen from a particular vantage.

In this indirect way, Mach's picture reveals what is sometimes referred to as the *transparency* of perceptual experience. It is as if experience itself is transparent.[43] When we try to describe it, we see through it, as it were, to the world. This is at once an important fact about visual phenomenology, and also an obstacle to phenomenology, at least construed in a particular way. The important fact is that perceptual experience—when we adapt a "natural attitude" and take our experience at face value—presents itself to us as a mode of awareness of *the world*. The obstacle to phenomenology is that the transparency of experience makes it seem puzzling how we can ever make experience itself the object of our inquiry. This is an important point, and we return to it later in the book (in section 5.5).

The transparency of experience is not an obstacle to phenomenology properly conceived. But it does show that we misconceive phenomenology if we think of it as concerned with the structure of the visual field.

We experience the world as unbounded and densely detailed because we do not inhabit a domain of visual snapshot-like fixations. When we hold our gaze fixed in that way, we do not look around, and insofar as we do not look around, we do not see. Vision is active; it is an active exploration of the world.

2.10   Active Perception

When we see, we do not represent the whole scene in consciousness all at once. Visual experiences do not present the scene in the way that a photograph does. In fact, seeing is much more like touching than it is like depicting. Consider the bottle again, which you touch with eyes closed. The bottle is there in your hands. By moving your hands, by palpation, you encounter its shape. The bottle as a whole is present to you, not because you now represent it in the sense of having an internal model of it, but in the sense that you now understand the way in which it structures and controls your movements, and so your sensory stimulation. The content of your tactile experience is enacted by your exploratory hand movements. You perceive the bottle tactilely by means of a temporally extended process of directed finger and hand movements.

Vision acquires content in exactly this way. You aren't given the visual world all at once. You are *in* the world, and through skillful visual probing—what Merleau-Ponty called "palpation with the eyes"—you bring yourself into contact with it. You discern its structure and so, in *that* sense, represent it. Vision is touch-like. Like touch, vision is *active*. You perceive the scene not all at once, in a flash. You move your eyes around the scene the way you move your hands about the bottle. As in touch, the content of visual experience is not given all at once. We gain content by looking around just as we gain tactile content by moving our hands. You enact your perceptual content, through the activity of skillful looking.

3 Enacting Content

Nothing that is seen is perceived at once in its entirety.
—Euclid

To localize an object simply means to represent to oneself the movements that would be necessary to reach it.
—H. Poincaré

It is only because we are active beings that our world is bigger than the content of our actual experience.
—C. I. Lewis

3.1 Spatial Content

We are not given the visual world all at once as in a picture; we must reach out and grasp the detail (as it were) by movements of our eyes and head. We possess the sensorimotor knowledge to be effective in our exploration. It is this mastery that is the basis of our sense of the presence to vision of what is in fact beyond our reach. It is this mastery that is the basis of perceptual content.

In this chapter I consider the ways perceptual experience acquires *spatial* content due to the perceiver's implicit understanding of the way sensory stimulation varies as a result of movement.

3.2 On What We See

It is a basic fact about perception that opaque, solid objects, when seen, have visible and invisible parts (Koenderink 1984b). From a given position, you can only see part of the surface of an object. Suppose, for example, that there is a tomato on the table in front of you. The facing side (facet) of the tomato itself is interposed between you and the far side and underneath (as well as the insides) of the tomato. You can only see part of the tomato's surface.

Some philosophers have challenged this basic fact about visual perspective. Thompson Clarke (1965), for example, proposes that seeing a tomato is like nibbling a piece of cheese. When you nibble a piece of cheese, you thereby nibble *it*, not merely a part of it. And so with seeing. It is only under special circumstances, according to Clarke, that you can be said, in looking at a tomato, to be seeing only a part of it. This would be natural to say, for example, if the part of the tomato you see were detached from the rest of the tomato. In the absence, however, of a feature of the situation that leads you thus attentively to focus selectively on a part of the tomato, when you look at a tomato, what you see is not part of it (the facing surface), but *it*.

Clarke is certainly right that in most circumstances in which you would naturally say that you see a tomato it would be odd to say that, really, you see only a part of its surface. But the general claim—that it is false that you only see part of the tomato when you look at it—is unconvincing. Consider that when you nibble a piece of cheese, you really do nibble only a part of the cheese, not the whole of it. If you were to cut off the part you nibbled, you'd be left with an unnibbled piece of cheese. And so, likewise, when you turn the tomato around, you get to see facets of the tomato that had been hidden from view.

A deeper objection to the claim that when you see a tomato, you only really see a part of its surface is phenomenological. You would misdescribe the visual experience of a solid, voluminous item of fruit, the tomato, if you were to describe it as an experience as of a bit of surface. Experiencing a bit of surface isn't like experiencing a solid thing. If you take your experience at face value, that is, as it presents itself to you, then you must describe it as an experience of, say, an ovoid solid object with a furrow (Koenderink 1984b).

This objection, first made by P. F. Strawson (1979), is well taken. However, it doesn't challenge the basic perspectival fact we are considering. Indeed, precisely what makes the perspectival fact interesting is a further point to which Strawson calls attention: Despite the fact that you can only see part of the object's surface, in looking at it we enjoy an experience as of a voluminous solid.

This is an example of what, in chapter 2, I called the problem of perceptual presence. We can draw here on the line of argument presented there. What explains the fact that you experience the tomato as voluminous and three-dimensionally extended, is that, for example, in looking at the tomato, you implicitly take it that were you to move your eyes a bit to the left or right, or up or down, you would bring previously hidden or obscured parts of the tomato into view. Your perceptual experience of the tomato as voluminous depends on your tacit understanding of the ways its appearance (how it looks) depends on movement. You visually experience parts of the tomato that, strictly speaking, you do not see, because you understand, implicitly, that your sensory relation to those parts is mediated by familiar patterns of sensorimotor dependence.

You do not merely experience the tomato as three-dimensionally extended, you experience it as possessing that characteristically tomato-like ovoid-with-a-furrow shape. We need to extend the enactive account somehow to explain how an encounter with the facing side of the tomato can serve as the basis for the experience of its shape.

Consider, first, the simple case of a cube. A cube has six sides or facets; there are twelve edges and eight vertices. You can never see more than three facets from a single point of view. Following Koenderink (1984b), we can call the aspect of the cube available from a vantage point the visible facets of the cube from that vantage point. As you move around the cube, its aspect changes dramatically. Facets come into view while others disappear. The *visual potential* of a cube (at least with respect to shape) is the way its aspect changes as a result of movement (of the cube itself, or of the perceiver around the cube). Any movement determines a set of changes in perceived aspect; any set of changes in perceived aspects determines equivalence classes of possible movements.

When you see the cube from a particular vantage point, you encounter its aspect from that vantage point. As you move with respect to the cube, you learn how its aspect changes as you move—that is, you encounter its visual potential. To encounter its visual potential is thus to encounter its actual shape. When you experience an object as cubical merely on the basis of its aspect, you do so because you bring to bear, in this experience, your sensorimotor knowledge of the relation between changes in cube aspects and movement. To experience the figure as a cube, on the basis of how it looks, is to understand *how* its look changes as you move.

Tomatoes, no less than cubes, have determinate visual potentials, or, as we can think of the visual potential, sensorimotor profiles. The sensorimotor profile of an object is the way its appearance changes as you move with respect to it (strictly speaking, it is the way sensory stimulation varies as you move). All solid, opaque objects have sensorimotor profiles in just this sense. As we get to more complicated forms, such as animal bodies, plants, and so forth, the mathematics needed to determine the sensorimotor profile of an object gets more complicated. Our visual perceptual skills, however, are that sophisticated, encompassing these complex (but ultimately manageable) relationships.

In this way the enactive approach explains the perceptual presence of shape, that is, how visual experience can present objects to us as having three-dimensionality, volume, and shape. The approach reconciles the dueling phenomenological facts noted previously: that perceptual experience represents the world as voluminous, and so forth, *and* that you cannot see anything in front of which an opaque surface is placed.

This sort of apparent conflict is rife in the domain of perceptual experience. For example, you see a round (i.e., circular) plate from an oblique angle; it looks elliptical to you, even though you can see that it is round (can experience it *as* round).[1] Some philosophers will not scruple to acknowledge commonplaces such as this. It is just not true that the plate looks elliptical, they will say. But how can we take this seriously? Certainly it is the case that we wouldn't be likely to judge the plate to be elliptical, on the basis of how it looks. Nor is it likely that we would say that it looks elliptical. But surely it does look elliptical from here!

Moreover, it's no accident that the circular plate looks elliptical. Elliptical is just how circular plates viewed from an angle look. Indeed, we experience the plate *as circular* precisely because we encounter its elliptical look from here, and we understand the transformations the elliptical apparent shape (aspect) would undergo as we move. That is, we understand that its elliptical look depends on our spatial relation to it, a relation that is modulated by movement. When you move with respect to a plate, its profile changes. We grasp the way its profile changes as we move, and we encounter the actual shape of the plate in thus bringing to bear our sensorimotor understanding. Our appreciation of its actual shape consists in our perception of its profile and our understanding of the way the profile, or apparent shape, depends on movement. We may say, in a case such as this, that we are able to experience the shape of the plate, to see it, because we grasp, implicitly, the sensorimotor profile of the plate. Our grasp of the plate's sensorimotor profile makes its shape available in experience.

Let's consider a different example: You see two trees and you see that they are roughly the same size.[2] One of the trees is nearer to you. The nearer tree looks larger to you in the sense that it takes up more of your visual field. Here, as in the cases of the plate and the tomato, one wants to ask, how can one reconcile two apparently conflicting ways of describing what is seen? We experience the trees as both similar in size and different in size.

As with the tomato and the plate, the conflict is apparent. We see that the trees are the same size. But we see their sameness of size not *despite* the fact that they differ in their apparent sizes, but *because* they do. We see their sameness of size in the fact that they look to be of different sizes *from here*. The experience of the actual size of the tree depends on the implicit grasp of how the apparent size is fixed by your relation to the tree.

Size, shape, voluminousness, and distance are experienced by us thanks to our possession of sensorimotor knowledge. These are central examples of the way in which, according to the enactive view, perceptual experience acquires content thanks to the perceiver's sensorimotor understanding.

3.3   The Reality of Appearances

Is perception direct? Many philosophers and perceptual psychologists have defended the idea that the true objects of perceptual experience are not things (events, etc.) in the world, but rather are mental items or "sense data." (See Noë 2002d for a brief review of this topic.) When we describe our experience in terms of tomatoes and plates and trees, for example, we go beyond what is, strictly speaking, given to us in experience (Ayer 1973). This widespread idea about the nature of perception is associated with a general epistemological and metaphysical standpoint known as phenomenalism. According to phenomenalism, objects are (in John Stuart Mill's excellent phrase) "permanent possibilities of sensation"; they are, in a more recent idiom, "logical constructions" of sense data.

Phenomenalism is a thorn in philosophy's side. It is hard to believe that it could be true. But it can also seem as if it must be true. According to one forcible line of argument on its behalf known as the *argument from illusion* (Ayer, 1995, 1973), what we experience are not the things we might naïvely think, but rather (at best) mental stand-ins for such things. The reasoning is as follows: It is impossible to tell, on the basis of your current experience, whether you are actually seeing what you think you see, or merely hallucinating it. It follows that the presence or absence of the putative object of perception can make no difference to your current experience. Whatever you are aware of, then, when you have the experience, it can't be the objects perceivers naïvely think they are aware of.

This argument has been criticized by numerous philosophers over the years. Austin (1962), for example, argued that from the fact that we can't tell, by reflecting on our experience, that our experience is veridical, it does not follow that a veridical experience is indistinguishable from a nonveridical one. You may not be able to tell the difference between a song by the Rolling Stones and one by Uncle Tupelo. That doesn't mean there isn't a difference. In general, there is a difference between how things look or sound, say, and how they look or sound *to one*. By the same token, looking like a Rembrandt *to one* may not be very strong evidence that the picture actually *looks like* a Rembrandt.[3] If this is right, then we must leave open the possibility that there are differences between veridical and nonveridical experiences, differences that depend precisely on the fact that in one case, but not the other, the experience is actually an experience of, say, a tomato (as argued by Snowdon [1980–1981] and McDowell [1982, 1986]; see also Putnam 1999, especially 152–153).

It is worth noting, as an aside, that there usually are differences in what it is like to have an experience and what it is like to have a nonveridical experience with "the same" content (Austin 1962; Putnam 1999). Austin noticed this when he observed that the experience of a bent-looking straight stick in a beaker of water is altogether unlike the experience of a bent stick. For one thing, there is the beaker of water (Austin 1962)! But the tendency to misdescribe the character of nonveridical experiences is surprisingly widespread, as I discussed in section 2.8. Filling in at the blind spot provides an example: We *mis*describe the experience of bar in figure 2.2 as the experience of a gapless bar; rather, the experience is better described as one in which we fail to perceive the break because it is blocked from view by the blind spot. I made a similar point about the illusory contours in figures 2.7. Granted, we naturally say here that "there appear to be contours where in fact there are none." The appearance of the illusory contours in figure 2.7, however, as discussed in section 2.8, is *not* qualitatively identical to the appearance of genuine contours, as illustrated by comparison with figure 2.8.

Other optical illusions—for example, the rectangular appearance of the trapezoidal Ames room[4]—are an artifact of a particular viewing position. It is only by requiring a subject to remain fixed that there is any tendency to *mis*perceive the room (Gibson 1979). In a more full-blooded sense, then, the illusory rectangular room doesn't look rectangular at all!

The simple point that these examples suggest is that we ought to be more cautious in describing the content of our experience of visual illusions. The more subtle point is this: Austin is right that, in general, from the fact that we are disposed, reasonably and in good faith, to describe an illusory experience as an experience of an F, say, it doesn't follow that the experience is *qualitatively indistinguishable* from a veridical experience of an F (Putnam 1999, 153). (I return to this issue in chapter 7.)

The deepest objection to the sense-datum approach, and to the associated phenomenalism, is that of P. F. Strawson (1979), mentioned earlier. It is not the case that we "go beyond" what is strictly given in our experience when we describe our experience as an experience of a round, three-dimensional solid item of fruit (as Ayer [1973] had suggested). To describe experience in sense-datum terms is to hold off from taking experience at face value; it is to "step back" from experience as it normally presents itself to us. The experience is, when we take it at face value, precisely an experience as of, say, a solid item of fruit on the table. It is not an experience as of a round, red sense datum. Our experiences purport to present the world to us.

These are important criticisms of the sense-datum theory. Let us assume, for the sake of argument, that they are successful; they count against the sense-datum theory and phenomenalism. However, as suggested earlier, they leave unscathed what is really the sense-datum theory's core idea: that perceiving is a way of finding out how things are from how they look or sound or, more generally, appear. This core idea—the truth in the sense-datum theory—can be divorced from the epistemologically and metaphysically threatening idea of phenomenalism. Looks, sounds, feels—appearances generally—are perceptually basic. They are the basis of our perceptual understanding of the world. Perception has two aspects or moments: We find out about appearances, and in finding out about appearances we find out about (come into contact with) the world.

Peacocke (1983) has attempted to do justice to the intuition that seeing is a two-step process—that it is, in the first instance, a mode of awareness of how things look—without succumbing to the mistakes of the sense-datum theory. It will prove instructive to consider his position.

According to Peacocke, when you have a visual experience—say, the experience with the content that geese are flying overhead—there is some way the visual experience presents the world to you as being. A complete description of the visual experience must mention this *representational content*. But in addition to its representational features, Peacocke argues, perceptual experience also possesses qualitative or sensational features that are not features of the way the experience represents things as being. Sensational properties of experience are features of what it is like to have an experience that are not features the experience represents the environment as exhibiting. (Sensational properties are often called 'qualia' in the philosophical literature.)

The argument for sensational properties goes like this. One can see, for example, that two trees are the same size, even as one also sees that one tree (the nearer one) looks larger than the other (the farther one) in the sense that it takes up more of the visual field. "Since," as Peacocke writes, "no veridical experience can represent one tree as larger than another and also as the same size as the other," it would seem, he concludes, that "size in the visual field" is a nonrepresentational feature of the experience (Peacocke 1983, 12). It is a sensational property.

Exactly similar points can be made, mutatis mutandis, about shape and, as Peacocke notes, color (see Peacocke 1983, 12–13).

This reasoning appears to be unsound. The fact that no veridical experience can represent one tree as larger than another and also as the same size as the other, does not entail that "size in the visual field" is a sensational property of experience.

We can distinguish size and apparent size, or size and *how things look with respect to size from here* ("size in the visual field"). Size in the visual field is a distinct property from size. It corresponds to the size of the patch that one must fill in on a given plane perpendicular to the line of sight in order to perfectly occlude an object from view. So long as you specify the plane as located, say, at some distance in front of the perceiver, how things look with respect to size can be recognized to be a perfectly definite property *of the scene* (Armstrong 1961; Harman 1990). Let us call this property the perspectival size of an object.[5]

One can distinguish shape and perspectival shape in the same way. We can speak, more generally then, of perspectival properties (or P-properties). P-properties are themselves *objects of sight*, that is, things that we see. They are visible. From where you stand, you can see the P-shape of the plate, and you can distinguish this from its actual shape. And so, likewise, you can see the difference in P-size of the trees even though you also see that they are the same in size.

In normal life we tend to pay little attention to P-properties. Only in special circumstances (e.g., in the task of artistic rendering) do they become salient. With a little effort, we can become quite skilled in noticing and describing them. This does not mean that we are not perceptually sensitive to them, even when we fail to attend to them. (I return to this topic briefly in chapter 5.)

P-properties—the apparent shape and size of objects—are perfectly "real" or "objective." Indeed, the relation of P-shape and P-size to shape and size can be given by precise mathematical laws (e.g., the laws of linear perspective). Importantly, in order to characterize P-properties, there is no need to refer to sensations or feelings. P-properties are objective in the sense that they are determinate and that they do not depend on sensations or feelings.[6]

However, P-properties are relational. In particular, P-properties depend on relations between the perceiver's body and the perceived object (and also on conditions of illumination). P-properties are, in effect, relations between objects and their environment. That a plate has a given P-shape is a fact about the plate's shape, one determined by the plate's relation to the location of a perceiver, and to the ambient light. The P-shape is the shape of the patch needed to occlude the object on a plane perpendicular to the line of sight. The P-size of the trees is, in turn, a fact about how the trees look, with respect to size, from the location of the perceiver: It is identical to the size of a patch we can imagine drawn on the occlusion plane. If there is a mind/world divide (in a Cartesian sense, a divide between the mental interior and the nonmental outside), then P-properties are firmly on the world side of the divide. They depend on relations to perceivers, yes. But perceivers (at least their bodies) are also on the world side of the divide.

A further sense in which P-size (but not other P-properties) is relational is revealed when you consider that P-size is relative to a plane of occlusion. Because there are an infinite number of occlusion planes, one can only speak of *the* perspectival size of an object if one can specify a single occlusion plane. (In the next section I return to this point, which was brought to my attention by Peter Murray.) However there *is* a single apparent size of an object—namely, the unique way that an object looks with respect to size from a particular position. This is secured by phenomenology. Given this, there must be a plane (or perhaps a class of planes) on whose surface an occluding patch would correspond to the P-size of the object.

This last point directs us to amend what has been said about the status of P-properties. P-properties are real (or objective) in the sense that they do not depend, for their nature, either on what goes on in us (e.g., sensations), or on what we do. P-properties are properties of the environment. Nevertheless, P-properties are only available (visible, audible, etc.) to creatures with the right kind of sensorimotor apparatus (e.g., the right kind of bodies). Insofar as they are there *for us*, it is only owing to our natures as agents with sensorimotor skills. I turn to this issue in the next section.

3.4   Conditions on the Possibililty of the Experience of Appearances

The crux is that P-properties are not merely visible qualities, such as shape and size.[7] They are *looks* of things, their visual appearances. To see a circular plate from an angle, for example, is to see something with an elliptical P-shape, and it is to understand how that perspectival shape would vary as a function of one's (possible or actual) movements with respect to the perceived object. We see its circularity *in* the fact that it looks elliptical from here.[8] We can do this because we understand, implicitly, that circularity is given in the way *how things look with respect to shape* varies as a result of movement. This is an example of the way visual experience can acquire content thanks to our possession and exercise of sensorimotor skills. In the same vein, it is not an accident that trees of the same size, but at different distances, differ in their perspectival size. To see the actual size of a thing is to see how its perspectival size varies as we move.

According to the enactive view, to see a spatial feature such as the size or shape of an object is to explore the way the look of the object varies as we move; it is to keep track of movement-dependent changes in P-properties.

This idea is closely related to one of Gibson's. The actual shape and size are invariants we encounter when we explore visual variation produced by movement. Consider a simple example of Gibson's. As you move around a rectangular table, you perceive its varying trapezoidal perspectival shape. The perspectival shape varies as your spatial relation to the table varies. In this pattern of variation, however, there is invariance. Mathematically what is invariant is the relationship between the four angles and the four sides and their proportions (Gibson 1979). This invariance corresponds to the actual shape of the table. Active exploration of the occlusion structure presents you with the actual shape of the table. The invariant structure of reality unfolds in the active exploration of appearances.

In this way, we can appreciate the truth in that basic idea of the sense-datum view—that perception has two moments, the encounter with how things appear and the encounter with how things are. We experience the world by experiencing how it looks.

But this is no defense of phenomenalism, at least as this is usually understood. To appreciate why, consider these two points.

First, according to this enactive account of perception, looks are not mental entities. Looks are objective, environmental properties. They are relational, to be sure. But they are not relations between objects and the interior, sensational effects in us. Rather, they are relations among objects, the location of the perceiver's body, and illumination. Perception may be a mode of encountering how things are by encountering how they appear. But this encounter with how they appear is itself an encounter with the world. For how things appear is a matter of how things are in the world. What is encountered (or "given") in perception is not sensational qualities or sense data, but rather the world.

Second, perception, according to the enactive approach, is direct and noninferential. We don't conjecture or infer how things are from how they look. In actively encountering the way in which how things look varies with movement, we *directly* encounter how things are. The circularity of the plate is made manifest in the way the profile changes as a result of movement. My experience of the circularity *just is* my experience of the variation in its perspectival shape. Furthermore, one doesn't *think* that the plate is round on the basis of the evidence of the senses, for example, that it looks elliptical. One experiences its roundness through the mastery of its sensorimotor profile. One doesn't infer that the tomato is a three-dimensional whole. One experiences it as a whole insofar as one encounters it by the exercise of an appropriate battery of sensorimotor skills.

It's worth mentioning that this is compatible with the fact that perception is fallible. You may experience a plate as circular, thanks to its elliptical appearance, when in fact it is elliptical. This is the possibility that informs a set of fascinating psychological constructions by Ames in which one misperceives, say, a trapezoidal window as rectangular, or a distorted room as rectilinear (the Ames room), or a tangle of lines as a chair (Ittelson 1952; Gregory [1966] 1997, 177–181; Gombrich 1960–1961, 247–250). In cases such as this, one does not misperceive because one misjudges, although one may misjudge. Rather, one misperceives because one draws on the wrong sensorimotor skills and expectations. That in which the experienced rectangularity of the trapezoidal window frame consists is precisely the fact that you have a certain range of expectations about the effects of movement in respect of it.

Finally, experience can acquire content in this way only if experience is active and dynamic in the way that the enactive approach proposes. You *don't* encounter the rectangularity in the P-shape alone. You encounter rectangularity in the variation in P-shape as you move (or as objects move with respect to you). It is only by exploring (or by being able to explore) visual space that you encounter the circularity. It is in the possible changes in P-shape that the real shape is encountered. The claim is that by sampling the way appearances change as you move through this appearance space, we encounter the invariants. This was, in essence, Gibson's idea about the ambient optic array. For an active creature, exploration of the ambient optic array *reveals* the world; it uniquely specifies it.

It's worth calling attention to a way in which the phenomenalist is right, at least from the standpoint developed here. Phenomenalism treats objects as constructions of sense data, as we have seen. Objects, in Mill's phrase again, are permanent possibilities of sensation. This thesis is wrong as metaphysics, but it's nearly right as an account of perceptual content. It is because mobile perceivers gain access to variation in perspectival properties as they move about that the actual spatial properties of objects are made available to the subject for experience. The world is made available to us in a way that is determined by the fact that we occupy a tentative and shifting place within the world. All perception is perspectival in this way (even perception in nonvisual modalities such as touch).[9]

3.5 Experiencing Looks

I have argued that perceptual experience acquires spatial content—comes to represent the shape and size of things—thanks to our possession of a battery of sensorimotor skills. As we move and perceptually explore the environment, we encounter variation in how things look. This variation in looks reveals how things are. But what of the looks themselves, what of P-properties? Do we *see them* by seeing how *they* look? This would threaten to lead to infinite regress (after all, one would need to experience the looks of the looks in order to see how things are, and so on, ad infinitum). How can we explain the sensorimotor basis of our experience of the looks of things?

Looks are relations between objects of perception and the environment (perceiver locations, ambient light, etc.). To experience a look (to see a look) is to make use, in experience, of a particular sensorimotor profile; it is to draw on our repertoire of sensorimotor skills.

Let's begin with a simple case: the experience of an item (a bit of movement, a sound, whatever) as *off to the left*. To experience the item as off to the left is to experience the object as occupying a certain position in one's egocentric space. What position? Precisely a position such that, in order to point to the object, one would need to move one's hands and arm to the left, and such that, in order to get a better look at the object, one would need to turn one's head to the left, in such and such a way, and such that, in order to distance oneself from the thing, one would need to move one's body to the right. Here, "left" and "right" are used egocentrically, not to denote regions of space but to denote spatial regions thought of in relation to the perceiver's body.[10] To move to the left, in this sense, is to make a characteristic movement of one's body. To experience something as off to the left, is to experience it not merely as occupying a region of space, nor is it merely to experience it as standing in a spatial relation to one; it is to experience one's relation to it as mediated by certain kinds of possible movements. Egocentric space, as Evans (1982) has argued, is in this sense a kind of *behavioral* space, that is, a space defined by ways of moving and behavioral degrees of freedom. To put the idea in my terms: To experience an object as off the left is to experience it as standing in a relation to one which one grasps as constituted by patterns of sensorimotor dependence. To experience it as on the left is to experience it as necessitating or admitting (indeed, in some sense, as *affording*) various possibilities of sense-affecting movements.

Similar points can be made about the experience of motion (as has been discussed recently by Philip Pettit 2003b). To experience a ball, say, as moving toward you is not to have an experience of a special sort of quality (the "something's moving toward one"-quale), just as the experience of the item's being off to the left is not the experience of a special quality or sensation of leftness. When you experience the ball as moving toward you, you experience it, precisely, as such that, by moving, you would change the character of the way its appearance changes. Certainly, it is also true that you experience it as such that, if you don't move, it will hit you. Your experience of its motion is an experience of it as enabling the possibility of a range of characteristic stimulation altering movements. There are countless ways in which your experience of a certain type of motion draws on sensorimotor understanding. You understand, for example, that if you move, then your visual sense of the ball's movement will be affected; that if you shut your eyes, it won't *visually* seem to be moving. To experience the ball as moving in an arc is to experience it, precisely, as moving in such a way that to track it you would need to move your head in a characteristic way. The experience of a thing's movements depends on your understanding of the sorts of sensorimotor contingencies mediating your relation to the thing. (This sensorimotor understanding is in fact the ground of your possession of dispositions to respond to the presented object.)

It is important that the kind of sensorimotor knowledge whose possession enables you to grasp your spatial relation to things is practical, not theoretical. Evans (1982) makes this point. One may have no clue where a given region of space that is off to one's left is, even though one experiences something as being there. One can implicitly understand its location in one's behavior space without having any more sophisticated cognitive grasp of where it is (in absolute space). It takes no thought or intellectual skill to know that to bring the item off to the left better into view, you must turn your head to the left.

Consider an example of Evans's. When you hear a sound as being on the left, you don't need to *think* about which way to turn in order to orient toward the sound. Hearing it as being on the left is bundled, as it were, with the understanding that to turn to the left is to turn toward the sound (that doing so would increase the intensity of the relevant sound). You do need to think about how to maneuver a couch to squeeze it through a small passage. But you do not need, in the same way, to think about how to maneuver your body to squeeze it through the doorway. Just perceiving the doorway as having certain spatial qualities is perceiving it as enabling, requiring, or permitting certain kinds of movement with respect to it. With the sound, and the passage through the door, one is occupied with egocentric, behavioral space. With the couch and the small passage, one is concerned with geometry and absolute space. Only in the latter case, but not the former, would one need to think, calculate, and measure.

This account enables us to explain the experience of P-properties. The plate looks elliptical to me because, to indicate its shape, I can (and indeed, in some sense, *must*) move my hand in a characteristic manner. That is, to experience a thing as elliptical is precisely to experience it as occupying a particular kind of region in one's egocentric, sensorimotor space. To experience the P-size of the tree is to experience it as taking up a region in my visual field, a space I indicate with a certain gesture of my arm. In this way, my sensorimotor skill is drawn on to constitute my experience of the shape.

The P-size of the object is given precisely as *that region* to which I, for example, would point or reach (etc.) if I wished to direct myself to the object. Great care is required here on two scores. First, I do not mean to be offering a definition of the experience of size, say, in terms of behavioral dispositions. Evans (1982) sometimes seems to offer such a behaviorist account, suggesting that the experience of something as off to the left consists, as it were by definition, precisely in the possession of certain behavioral dispositions to move with respect to the thing. My claim is not behaviorist in the way that Evans's appears to be. When we see a flicker on the right, we know—in a practical, implicit way—that movements of the eyes to the right bring (or would bring) the flicker better into view. The experience of the flicker as on the visual egocentric right consists not in our disposition to move in certain ways, but in our possession of a kind of practical knowledge of how *movement* would bring the thing into view. A different rule of sensorimotor contingency applies if the flicker occurs on the left. To experience it as on the left is to know that leftward movements of the eyes and head will bring it into the center of the visual field. Experience could not present itself to us as having spatial content in this way, if we did not possess the sensorimotor skills needed thus to modulate our relation to it in spatially relevant ways.

Second, I do not mean to be offering an account of the significance of sensory experience in terms of what we use that experience to do, for example, the guidance of movements, the avoidance of projectiles, and so forth. There is no question that experience can and does guide movement, but it is not the business of the enactive view to emphasize this humdrum fact. The enactive view (as stressed in chapter 1) proposes not that perceiving is *for* acting, but rather that perceiving is constituted by the exercise of a range of sensorimotor skills. In this setting, then, I do not wish to argue that to experience something as having a certain (apparent, perspectival) shape is to experience it as affording a range of possible movements; rather, I want to suggest that one experiences it as having a certain P-shape, and so as affording possible movements, only insofar as, in encountering it, one is able to draw on one's appreciation of the sensorimotor patterns mediating (or that might be mediating) your relation to it.[11] How you appreciate it as being is constituted by the sensorimotor knowledge you bring to bear in your encounter with it.

According to the enactive view I am defending here, to experience something as elliptical is to perceive it as thus occupying a position in one's *sensorimotor* space. Only someone who understands, implicitly, that turning the eyes to the left brings an item on the left into view, can be said to experience something as *on the left*. Someone with this knowledge can enjoy the corresponding experiences.

How things look *to me* is constrained by my sensorimotor knowledge. It is my possession of basic sensorimotor skills (which include the abilities to move and point and the dispositions to respond by turning and ducking, and the like) that enables my experience to acquire *visual* content at all. With further sensorimotor knowledge, my perceptual experience acquires full-blown perceptual content.

Note that there is nothing in this account to rule out the capacity of people who are behaviorally limited from having experiences of spatial looks. To experience a thing as being on the left is to experience it as occupying a relation to one defined by possibilities of movement. This is compatible with its being the case that someone who is incapable of movement could have perceptual experience as of something on the left. What is ruled out is the possibility of someone who lacked all sensorimotor comprehension having experiences with spatial content (or, for that matter, any content).

3.6 Inverting Goggles, Revisited

When you put on inverting lenses, you experience not an inversion of content, but a disruption or disorganization of content. As discussed in chapter 1, this "experiential blindness" is to be expected from the enactive standpoint. Mere sensory stimulation in the absence of an understanding of the way stimulation is modulated by movement does not rise to the level of perceptual experience. For stimulation to be genuinely perceptual—that is, for it to be the case that in being stimulated you are also made perceptually aware of properties and states of affairs around you—you need sensorimotor knowledge. The effect of putting on the goggles is, precisely, to alter sensorimotor laws. Perceptual adaptation to inverting goggles is, therefore, in the first instance, a process whereby sensorimotor understanding, and with it perceptual content, is restored.

Let's look a bit more closely at the details of perceptual adaptation to reversing goggles. As noted in chapter 1, work by Kohler ([1951] 1964) and Taylor (1962) suggests that perceptual adaptation has three distinct stages. First, there's the initial experiential blindness, as discussed in this chapter, and in chapter 1. We can refer to the experience of content-inverted perceptual experience as the second stage of adaptation to the goggles. Once you get somewhat accustomed to the lenses, objects on the left will look to you as if they are on the right, and vice versa. The enactive view can explain the occurrence of this content inversion. Movements of the eyes to the left produce the sensorimotor consequences previously associated with an object on the right, and vice versa. Previously the experience of "leftness" consisted precisely in, say, your grasp of the way in which movements of the body affect your relation to the object on the left. To say that the object on the left looks as if it is on the right is to say that you implicitly take your relation to the object on the left to be that normally characterized by your relation to one on the right. For example, to reach out "to the left," you naturally move your hand in a rightward direction. To avoid a blow to the face coming from the right, you will naturally tend to move *to the right*. You acquire content by misassigning sensorimotor significance to your visual stimulation.

The third and final stage of adaptation is the stage at which the content of perceptual experience "veridicalizes" itself. The object on the left now looks, as it should, as if it is on the left, and objects on the right look as if they are on the right. This is so despite the fact that the left object stimulates parts of the retina and visual cortex that would normally be stimulated by objects on the right side of the visual field. This is genuine *perceptual plasticity*, that is, the transformation of perceptual content.

From the standpoint of the enactive view, it is not difficult to understand this righting or reinversion of perceptual content. An object is experienced *as on the left* when one takes one's relation to it to be mediated by the appropriate sensorimotor contingencies. Perceptual adaptation, from the enactive standpoint, is a process of learning to apply the appropriate sensorimotor knowledge. Once this is accomplished, content is refashioned. Veridicality is restored.

It is significant that perceptual adaptation is achieved only by individuals who *actively* interact with their environments. Taylor's subjects, for example, were made to engage in difficult sensorimotor tasks (welding, bike riding, etc.). This is not surprising from the standpoint of the enactive approach, for it is precisely through active movement that one is able to test sensorimotor hypotheses. Somewhat more surprisingly, however, is the fact that adaptation tends to be task-specific. Content may veridicalize for bike riding, say, but not for reading. Content may be reinverted sufficiently to enable you to bike around; nevertheless, when you bike past a row of shops, the writing on the store windows looks left-right reversed. A bit of reflection suffices to demonstrate that this "modular" pattern to adaptation isn't really all that surprising. It is not surprising that sensorimotor skills do not initially generalize readily across radically different tasks.

This kind of interpretation of the goggles experiments has been challenged by Harris (1965, 1980).[12] He denies that the experiments support the claim that there is genuine visual plasticity. According to Harris, there is no reinversion of perceptual content. There is merely an illusion of reinversion. The illusion that reinversion occurs, according to Harris, has two main sources. First, perceivers *get used* to the inverted visual world. Experiences with inverted content thus lose their strangeness. Just as it is possible, through practice and familiarity, to come to read mirror-reversed writing as if it were normal, so, after the passage of time, the left-right reversal of content comes to seem normal. Second, and more important for our purposes, one's sense of movement (kinesthesis) and body position (proprioception) come to adapt to vision.

To appreciate the significance of this second point, consider that the second stage of adaptation to inverting goggles produces an intermodal conflict between vision and proprioception/kinesthesis. You look down at your feet. Your left foot looks as if it is on the right, but it *feels* as if it is on the left. This conflict is certainly a source of your sense of the strangeness. You look at your left hand. It looks as if it is on the right, but it feels as if it is on the left. Now imagine that you reach to pick up on object on the left. It looks as if it is on the right. So you reach to the right. Your hand looks as though it is reaching to the left, not the right, where the object appears to be located. So you move your hand more to the right, which adds to your sensory confusion.

Perceptual adaptation, according to Harris (at what I am calling the third stage), consists in the resolution of the conflict between proprioception/kinesthesis and vision in favor of vision. Now your left arm not only looks as if it is on the right, but comes to *feel* as if it is on the right as well. Your left foot not only looks to be on the right, but feels as if it is too. This has the following effect: Let's say you want to pick up the coffee on your left. It looks to you as if it is on the right. So you reach out for it with your left hand because that hand feels to you as if it is on the right. And you extend your left hand to the left, in the direction that now looks and feels as if it is on the right. Because the cup is actually on your left, you succeed in picking it up. Your visual experience is still reversed. Nothing has changed; there is no genuine perceptual reversal or plasticity. But you have accommodated to your reversal and, with practice, so Harris suggests, will stop noticing it. Your sense of movement and your position accommodate to your visual experience, and the result is that you are able to move around and act appropriately in your environment. Things feel normal even though your visual content is still inverted.

Harris's claims about perceptual reversal present the enactive view with an important challenge. For Harris makes the case that the visual experience of space is independent of facts about a perceiver's sensorimotor skills or dispositions to move. Behavioral facts contribute to the *illusion* of perceptual reinversion, but their obtaining doesn't make it the case that there is any such inversion. Harris believes that facts about the spatial content of perceptual experience are independent of what you do and also of what you believe (on the basis of introspection) about your own experience. The problem of space is very like that which arises in discussions of color experience and the inverted spectrum hypothesis. It will be helpful to explore this comparison.

Could it be the case that an individual has color experiences that are undetectably inverted relative to ours in the sense that yellow things look to him or her the way blue things look to us, and red things look to him or her they way green things look to us? Because we would all agree in what we call "red" and "yellow" (etc.), this difference in our experience would never show itself in our behavior. (This "inverted spectrum hypothesis" has been explored by Shoemaker [1982], Block [1990], and Palmer [1999b], among others). This hypothesis raises similar issues to a "spatial inversion hypothesis." Might a person's spatial experience be systematically, but undetectably, inverted relative to ours? Such a one would experience left-sidedness as we experience rightsidedness (and vice versa), but would agree with us in referring to this property as leftsidedness. In the color case, the strongest arguments ask us to consider the possibility in the first person. At stage 1, I am inverted. At stage 2, I get used to the inversion. I realize things now look color-inverted compared to the way they used to look, and I use this knowledge to guide my correct use of words. I get really good at acting normal. At stage 3, I suffer amnesia and forget that things ever looked different. The point of this thought experiment is that it suggests a reason to believe that things are now different with me with respect to my color experience, even though I am now unable to report these differences.

Harris's analysis of the inverting goggles experiments treats them as raising just this kind of issue. His claim is that we get so familiar with acting and talking and getting along with our spatially inverted visual experiences that we, in effect, come to forget that our experience is inverted. We even go so far as to report that things are back to normal. In fact, our experience remains as inverted as ever.

Whether the inverted spectrum hypothesis is altogether coherent is debatable.[13] I draw the comparison between spatial and color vision here in order to set out in clear relief the burden and significance of Harris's claim. Whatever we say about the color case, I find it highly implausible that we have any grip whatsoever on spatial content apart from perceivers' sensorimotor skills. As suggested in section 3.5, it is unclear what one's experience of a sound's coming from the egocentric right, say, could consist in apart from the perceiver's practical understanding that to move the eyes to the right is to move them to the source of the sound.[14]

Given this, it is tempting to suggest that there is a way of interpreting Harris's argument according to which it is, in effect, an argument *for* the enactive view. Perceptual adaptation may indeed be a process whereby the relation among visual stimulation and proprioceptive and kinesthetic information are made to cohere. But that's just to say that *visual* content is constituted by these relationships. Harris himself comes close to suggesting this when he writes: "So many visual judgments and visually guided behaviors are affected [by processes of adaptation] that one *could* talk about a modification of visual perception, as long as one bears in mind that here too what is actually modified is the interpretation of nonvisual information about positions of body parts" (1980, 113). Harris thinks we should keep clearly in the mind the fact that adaptation isn't *visual*, but has to do with information about "the interpretation of nonvisual information about positions of body parts." But maybe this is precisely what the *visual* transformation of spatial content consists in? If this is right, then it sheds light on the mechanisms of adaptation. One of the triggers for adaptation is the attempt of the brain to make sense of intermodal conflict among vision, proprioception, and kinesthesis.

For these reasons, I am skeptical of Harris's analysis. There are other problems with the position that deserve mention.

Consider, to start, the fact that Harris's view seems to presuppose a strong asymmetry among vision and proprioception and kinesthesis that is, on the face of it, puzzling. What is it about vision, on Harris's view, that prevents visual plasticity, but that allows proprioceptive and kinesthetic plasticity? On the enactive view, each of these modalities is on the same footing; their character is determined by patterns of sensorimotor integration. Moreover, on the enactive view, one should expect that visual content requires integration with kinesthesis and proprioception; after all, visual content depends on the sensory effects of movement. But by the same token, it is not particularly surprising that kinesthesis and proprioception depend on vision (and on other modalities). This is what we do find: The hand on the left (at the second stage of adaptation to the goggles) comes to *feel* as if it is on the right because its movements provoke visual stimulation previously associated with an object on the right.

Indeed, according to the enactive view, the hand on the left feels like *my* hand—that is, an animate, feeling part of me—only because of the role it plays as a sensorimotor nexus of movement and sensory stimulation. Given the right sort of integration in a sensorimotor nexus even a non-attached (e.g., prosthetic) hand could come to feel like *my* hand.[15]

Second, more generally, it is unclear how to make sense of the basis of spatial content in vision on Harris's approach. Is it Harris's view that what determines the visual experience of space are facts about patterns of retinal stimulation and retinotopic neural representations in visual thalmus and visual cortex? But then what is it, we can ask, about the intrinsic character of these neural structures or patterns thanks to which they give rise to experiences with one spatial content rather than another? As we noticed in chapter 2—in connection with the discussion of the homunculus fallacy—in general it is unacceptable to "read off" properties of internal neural systems from properties of corresponding perceptual experiences. There is no a priori reason why an experience of leftsidedness should have, as its neural substrate, a retinotopic neural structure. But if that is so, then it is unclear what explanatory work the existence of retinotopic maps is supposed to be performing.

For now I want to underscore that the enactive view offers an account of visual content that can bypass these thorny issues. Perceptual content is not fixed by neural structures, but by patterns of sensorimotor contingency and the animal's skillful mastery of them. Moreover—and this is significant—it does so in a way that squares with perceivers' reports on the character of their own experience. Harris's view, in contrast, necessitates treating perceptually adapted goggle wearers as deluded about the nature of their own experience.[16]

3.7 Berkeley and the Touch-Like Character of Seeing

Berkeley ([1709] 1975) held that touch is the only genuinely spatial sense. Touch alone, he seems to have thought, is intrinsically active, and it is only through physical movement that we directly encounter space. Other perceptual modalities acquire spatial content as a consequence of learned linkages with touch and movement.

My theme, in contrast, is the touch-like character of vision itself, by which I mean precisely the fact that vision too is intrinsically active. The enactive account of experience can be thought of as a generalization of Berkeley's account of the spatial content of touch to vision and the other sensory modalities. According to such a generalized view, spatial content is available to other modalities such as vision in just the way that it is available to touch, namely, in terms of its immediate significance for movement and action.

Why did Berkeley think touch was privileged in this way? He begins his investigation with the seeming paradox that we perceive spatial qualities such as distance even though they are imperceptible. He states: "It is plain that distance is in its own nature imperceptible, and yet it is perceived by sight" ([1709] 1975, §2).

Why is Berkeley so confident that we can immediately perceive spatial qualities by touch, that spatial qualities are, in effect, tactile? After all, you can't actually *touch* the distance separating you from an object, nor can its size or shape be taken in, immediately, in the way that hardness or even texture can be taken in. This suggests that there are *no* sensory ideas, tactile or otherwise, corresponding to spatial qualities such as distance or size in the way that there are sensory ideas corresponding to redness or hardness.

How then does tactile experience acquire spatial content? And what is it about the way it acquires this content that justifies claiming that spatial qualities are available to touch *immediately*?

Berkeley's proposal is compelling: Touch acquires content through movement. Touch is *intrinsically* active. It is, in effect, a kind of movement. And movement is intrinsically spatial in the sense that it unfolds in space and is thus mediated by space. Presumably Berkeley has in mind facts such as that the only way immediately to encounter spatial qualities like distance in perception is through movement. We cannot touch distance itself, but we can experience distance by reaching out and taking hold, or by getting up and moving. The distance of x is experienced by me in terms of, say, how many steps it would take to get to x, to bring x into contact with my hands. In experience what corresponds to distance is the implicit understanding of the quality and kind of movement needed to bring an object into contact. This is the idea captured succinctly by Poincaré in the epigraph to this chapter.

Similar points, as we have considered, hold for our experience of other spatial qualities such as shape and size. When you handle an object, you hold it and move your hands over its surface. You encounter its shape by encountering the way the object itself guides or impedes your movement. To experience a shape as spherical is to experience a characteristic uniformity as you move your hands, or move it about in your hands. The stimulation you receive is a function of your movements of the item in your hand, or the movement of your hands across your fingers. The shape is given, experientially, as a *sensorimotor* pattern.

Touch acquires spatial content—comes to represent spatial qualities—as a result of the ways touch is linked to movement and to our implicit understanding of the relevant tactile-motor dependencies governing our interaction with objects. Berkeley is right that touch is, in fact, a kind of movement. When a blind person explores a room by walking about in it and probing with his or her hands, he or she is perceiving by touch. Crucially, it is not only the use of the hands, but also the movement in and through the space in which the tactile activity consists. Very fine movements of the fingers and very gross wanderings across a landscape can each constitute exercises of the sense of touch. Touch, in all such cases, is movement. (At the very least, it is movement of something relative to the perceiver.) These Berkeleyan ideas form a theme, more recently, in the work of O'Shaughnessy (2000). He writes: "touch is in a certain respect the most important and certainly the most primordial of the senses. The reason is, that it is scarcely to be distinguished from the having of a body that can act in physical space" (O'Shaughnessy 2000, 658).

In comparison with touch, Berkeley thinks that sight and hearing provide spatial content only indirectly. For there are no direct linkages between seeing or hearing and moving. We *can* see spatial qualities such as distance and shape, but we cannot see them immediately (say, in the way we can see colors or feel textures). We see them by interpreting visual qualities as having spatial significance due to the fact that we have learned to associate visual qualities with tangible ideas about possibilities of movement. Bluntly put, we infer depth, distance, size, and three-dimensional shape from the qualities that we directly see.

This, then, is Berkeley's solution to the paradox of spatial perception. Visual experience acquires spatial content because we come to understand visual qualities as having *tangible* significance.

Berkeley is right that touch is intrinsically active. But why hold that touch is the only active sense modality? As we have stressed, the visual world is not given all at once, as in a picture. The presence of detail consists not in its representation now in consciousness, but in our implicit knowledge now that we can represent it in consciousness if we want, by moving the eyes or by turning our head. Our perceptual contact with the world consists, in large part, in our access to the world thanks to our possession of sensorimotor knowledge.

Here, no less than in the case of touch, spatial properties are available due to links to movement. In the domain of vision, as in that of touch, spatial properties present themselves to us as "permanent possibilities of movement." As you move around the rectangular object, its visible profile deforms and transforms itself. These deformations and transformations are reversible. Moreover, the rules governing the transformation are familiar, at least to someone who has learned the relevant laws of visuomotor contingency. How the item looks varies systematically as a function of your movements. Your experience of it *as* cubical consists in your implicit understanding of the fact that the relevant regularity is being observed.

Not only does the cubical quality of the object consist in the fact that our relation to it is mediated by certain patterns of sensorimotor dependence, but the visual perceptual character of the relation itself consists in the fact that blinking, turning away, and shutting off the lights affects your interaction with the object in ways that immediately disrupt these sensorimotor dependences. Stopping your ears, breathing in deeply, and putting on loud music have no similar effect on your relation to the object.

It is sometimes said that the main structural difference between seeing and touch comes out in the fact that touch requires that there be serial contact with things through time whereas sight allows one, as it were, to represent a spatial manifold, an array of objects at a distance from one's body in space. Even if we suppose this is true, caution is needed in assessing its significance. The culprit that threatens to mislead us here is the notion of perceptual content. To see how, consider an observation made by von Senden ([1932] 1960) in this connection. Von Senden had argued that, pace Berkeley, *vision* is the only true spatial sense, for only vision allows one to experience the spatial distribution of objects. Touch, in contrast, allows, at best, the representation of objects *through time*. One error in this view was identified by Evans (1982): It's a mistake to confuse (to put the point in Kant's idiom) the order of the perceptions themselves with the order and structure that is thus represented in the world. Touch may rely on exploration through time but that is no obstacle, says Evans, to the tactile representation of a spatial manifold.

Evans is right, but we can formulate the thought better like this: Touch can serve as the basis for experience of *a spatial* manifold of objects in just the same way that vision can. In having these experiences—tactile or visual—we can rightly take ourselves to be brought in contact with a spatial manifold.

However, a further misunderstanding lurks in the vicinity. From the fact that, in having the visual experience, we become aware of the spatial manifold, it does not follow that, as a matter of pure phenomenology, we can ever experience all the elements in the manifold in visual (or for that matter tactile) consciousness all at once. To suppose otherwise is to embrace the now discredited snapshot conception of perceptual phenomenology (see chapter 2), and it is to disregard the evidence of change blindness research (discussed in section 2.3).

This invites us to consider that vision may be more like touch than either von Senden or Berkeley had considered. Through attention, probing, and movements of the eyes, visual experience acquires content in much the same way that touch does. Vision, and touch, gain content through our skillful movements. We bring content to experience, by action. We *enact* content.

O'Shaughnessy (2000) may be right that there is a primacy to touch in the sense that touch, or at least touch *and* proprioception, would seem to be a prerequisite for movement and action, whereas vision, in comparison, is perhaps more of a luxury (an evolutionary latecomer). Nevertheless, only one capable of movement could enjoy visual experiences with spatial content. Moreover, the links between vision and movement are not mediated by touch, at least not in the way Berkeley thought.

3.8 Molyneux's Question

Berkeley believed that we can see spatial relations and properties only because we have learned to associate sight with tangible ideas of space. For this reason, he answered Molyneux's question negatively. Molyneux's famous question, posed to Locke (in a letter of March 2, 1694), then published in the second edition of Locke's *Essay Concerning Human Understanding* ([1689] 1975: II, ix, 8), was as follows:

Suppose a Man born blind, and now adult, and taught by his touch to distinguish between a Cube, and a Sphere of the same metal, and nighly of the same bigness, so as to tell, when he felt one and t'other, which is the Cube, which the Sphere. Suppose then the Cube and Sphere placed on a Table, and the Blind Man to be made to see. Quaere, Whether by his sight, before he touch'd them, he could now distinguish, and tell, which is the Globe, which the Cube.

Having been born blind, Berkeley reasoned, a person whose sight was restored later life, would be ignorant of the association between visible properties and tangible properties in which the spatial content of vision consists. As a result, Molyneux's man would not see that the item before him was, say, a sphere.

Almost every writer to discuss this question—and it has been, over the last few hundred years, a *hot* topic of discussion[17]—has followed Berkeley in answering it negatively. Only Leibniz, and more recently Gareth Evans, have answered Molyneux's question positively.

The enactive view, it will be clear, requires a positive answer to the question, at least subject to certain important qualifications. According to the enactive view, vision, no less than touch, is capable of representing spatial properties. Anyone who can see, therefore, will see spatial relations and properties. Given that Molyneux's man knows what spheres and cubes are on the basis of his tactile experience of the world, then he ought to be able to recognize those items by sight. (For practical reasons discussed in chapter 1, it is unlikely that Molyneux's man would be able to do this immediately after the surgery, for the surgery itself could not suffice to impart the required sensorimotor understanding.)

To explain, consider that what makes a negative answer to Molyneux's question seem unavoidable is the idea that there is nothing common to the way spatial properties look, feel, and sound. In one case we undergo tactile sensations, and in the other visual or auditory sensations. Only experience of the correlation of tactile, visual, and auditory sensations could enable one who had never seen, for example, to *see* a spatial quality he or she had previously only known through touch.

But the enactive view denies that we represent spatial properties in perception by correlating them with kinds of sensation. There is no *sensation* of roundness or distance, whether tactile, visual, or otherwise. When we experience something as a cube in perception, we do so because we recognize that its appearance varies (or would vary) as a result of movement, that it exhibits a specific sensorimotor profile. We represent spatial properties in perception not by having sensations with special, intrinsic qualities, but by appreciating a kind of structure or order in our sensations whatever their intrinsic quality.

This is the key to the enactive approach to Molyneux's question. The sensorimotor dependencies that govern the *seeing* of a cube certainly differ from those that govern the *touching* of one, that is, the ways cube appearances change as a function of movement is decidedly different for these two modalities. At an appropriate level of abstraction, however, these sensorimotor dependencies are isomorphic to each other, and it is *this* fact—rather than any fact about the quality of sensations, or their correlation—that explains how sight and touch can share a common spatial content. When you learn to represent spatial properties in touch, you come to learn the transmodal sensorimotor profiles of those spatial properties. Perceptual experience acquires spatial content thanks to the establishment of links between movement and sensory stimulation. At an appropriate level of abstraction, these are the same across the modalities.

We can illustrate this by means of a simple example. If something looks square, then one would need to move one's eyes or head in characteristic ways to look at each of the corners. One would have to move one's hands *the same way* (at the appropriate level of abstraction) to feel each corner.

Evans (1985) anticipated this conclusion. On his view, the common sensorimotor content of "looks square" and "feels square" is to be explained in terms of the fact that when we experience spatial qualities, we do so in terms of behavior space. But there is only *one* behavior space, even though we can move in it in different ways (e.g., by moving hands, or by moving eyes, etc.).

One might object that a positive answer to Molyneux's question is incompatible with the empirical evidence gathered from the study of cases of cataract surgery. As discussed in chapter 1, there is certainly reason to believe that postsurgical patients are unable to make correct perceptual judgments of shape and size. For example, Cheselden describes a boy who, after cataract removal surgery, is unable to determine visually the shape of a coin; he remarks that the coin appears to change its shape as it is rotated before him. Does this show that we need to answer Molyneux's question negatively?

I think not. For crucially, Cheselden's boy *did not* have his vision restored by the surgery. As discussed earlier, surgical removal of cataracts enables patients to receive relatively normal patterns of sensory impression. But, as I have stressed, normal sensory impressions are not sufficient for sight. To see one must understand the sensorimotor significance of these impressions. This necessary knowledge is absent in Cheselden's boy. He hasn't yet learned to see.

These considerations call into question whether it would ever be feasible to seek an empirical answer to Molyneux's question. Given that seeing requires sensorimotor knowledge—that is, learned links between visual stimulation and movement—we may be unable to find the sort of "sudden onset" vision that Molyneux's question imagines. An interesting case is that of sensory substitution systems such as TVSS (discussed in chapter 1, and also in O'Regan and Noë 2001a and Hurley and Noë 2003a,b). According to Bach-y-Rita (1972, 1983, 1984), blind subjects adapted to TVSS are able spontaneously to make judgments about spatial relations using tactile vision. They *perceive* the shapes and spatial relations of things even though they have never seen such things before. I turn to a more detailed discussion of this in section 3.9.

3.9   Gibson, Affordances, and the Ambient Optic Array

I have argued that the dynamic process of exploring appearance space constitutes a mode of contact with the environment. The process of exploring the environment is mediated by patterns of sensorimotor contingency. Another way to put this is that when we see, we experience the way the environment structures sensorimotor contingency. So, for example, it is the pattern of change in the P-shape of the table as one moves around it (a pattern in the structure of sensorimotor contingency) that informs the perceiver of the rectangularity of the table. It is precisely the way a ball, say, structures and limits one's hand movements that reveals the roundness of the ball. To learn how things are from how they look is to learn that the environment structures one's possibilities of movement and exploration. It is to discover the structure of sensorimotor contingencies.

Gibson famously held that the structure of light in the environment—what he called "the ambient optic array"—uniquely specifies the layout of surfaces in the environment (1979, chap. 5). The perceiver need only visually explore this ambient structure to find out how things are. Perception, according to Gibson, involves the "direct pickup" of information about the environment in the ambient light (1979, chap. 14). This led Fodor and Pylyshyn (1981) to argue that Gibson fails to break with the inferentialist assumptions of the so-called establishment.[18] For Gibson, no less than for traditional theorists, Fodor and Pylyshyn argue, we must have a more immediate epistemic relationship to light than we do to the environment the light specifies (Fodor and Pylyshyn 1981, 165–168).[19] What is "picked up directly," according to Fodor and Pylyshyn, is not how things are in the environment, but how they are with the light. Whether you call it inference or not, perception is mediated by a complex cognitive process whereby we recover facts about the layout from the information available in the light itself.

Gibson (1979) laid great stress on the fact that light, as it concerns ecological optics, is not the light of the physicist. Physical problems about light pertain to its nature as radiant energy traveling in waves or packets and to the laws governing its behavior. Ecological optics, in contrast, is concerned with ambient light, that is, with light as it fills space and interacts with the cluttered environment of the animal. Gibson criticizes traditional visual theory for failing to make this distinction. For Gibson, visual science must think of light—what he calls the ambient optic array—as providing information for the animal (not for the receptor).

I propose that we interpret the ambient optic array as the structured space of appearances. The ambient optic array, simply put, is how things look from here in these conditions. The sense of the Gibsonian claim that the ambient optic array specifies the environment (unlike the pattern of irradiation on the retina), is that how things look from here in these conditions specifies how they are, or rather, it does so for a suitably knowledgeable animal, one in possession of and ready to apply sensorimotor skill. That how things look specifies how things are is a substantive empirical claim. Ecological optics, on this view, seeks to investigate precisely the mechanisms by means of which the structure of appearances is uniquely determined by environmental layout.

This enables us to see the error of Fodor and Pylyshyn's criticism. First, there is an important sense in which it is false that, insofar as we see, we have a more direct epistemic relation to light than we do to the world that is illuminated by light. If we think of light the way the physicist does (e.g., as packets of energy), then, insofar as we see, it is not obvious that we have *any* epistemic relation to light. We see light sources (e.g., the sun, lightbulbs), and we see that which is illuminated by light. We do not see the light itself (Gibson 1979). But second, it is true that, in Gibson's view, as I am reconstructing it, it is awareness of the ambient optic array that provides the basis for our awareness of the environment. That is, we learn how things are by discovering their visual appearances. But visual appearances fall squarely on the world side of the mind/world divide. The active exploration of how things look (an aspect of reality) constitutes our very contact with how things are apart from how they look.

All this sheds light on the Gibsonian notion of an affordance (Gibson 1979, chap. 8). According to Gibson, the environment consists not only of surfaces and objects, but of "affordances." Things in the environment, and properties of the environment, offer or *afford* the animal opportunities to do things (find shelter, climb up, hide under, etc.). According to Gibson, information in the ambient optic array specifies not only properties of the layout of the environment, but also environmental affordances. We can directly perceive not only that there is a horizontal surface, but that there is something that affords support. When you see a tree, you not only directly perceive a tree, but you directly perceive something up which you can climb. Gibson took this feature of his theory to be quite radical, for it suggested that we directly perceive meaning and value in the world; we do not impose meaning and value on the world.

Gibson's view can now be usefully reformulated in the context of the enactive approach. To perceive, according to the view being developed here, is to perceive structure in sensorimotor contingencies. To see that something is flat is precisely to see it as giving rise to certain possibilities of sensorimotor contingency. To feel a surface as flat is precisely to perceive it as impeding or shaping one's possibilities of movement. We can put the point picturesquely by saying that when we perceive, we perceive in an idiom of possibilities for movement. This lends credence to Gibson's idea of affordances. To perceive is (among other things) to learn how the environment structures one's possibilities for movement and so it is, thereby, to experience possibilities of movement and action afforded by the environment. Gibson's theory, and this is plausible, is that we don't see the flatness and then interpret it as suitable for climbing upon. To see it as flat is to see it as making available possibilities for movement. To see it as flat is to see it, directly, as affording certain possibilities.

Affordances are animal-relative, depending, for example, on the size and shape of the animal. It is worth noting that they are also skill-relative. To give an example, a good hitter in baseball is someone for whom a thrown pitch affords certain possibilities of movement. The excellence of a hitter does not consist primarily in having excellent vision. But it may very well consist in the mastery of sensorimotor skills, the possession of which enables a situation to afford an opportunity for action not otherwise available.

According to the enactive view, there is a sense, then, in which *all* objects of sight (indeed, all objects of perception) are affordances. To experience a property is, among other things, to grasp its sensorimotor profile. It is to experience the object as determining possibilities of and for movement.

3.10   What Is a Sensory Modality?

Philosophers may be attracted to *the qualia theory*, according to which sensory modalities differ qualitatively. Seeing is different from touching, on this approach, because there are introspectibly accessible differences between experiences of seeing and touching. In favor of the qualia theory is the fact that perceivers can usually tell (but not always) whether they are seeing something, or feeling it. One might worry however—as Grice (1962) did—whether introspection can serve in this way in an account of the modalities. Grice held that the (putative) transparency of experience—the fact that when you turn your attention to your experience itself, you end up reflecting on *what* is experienced, rather than on the experience— suggests that introspection can't deliver the goods the qualia theory needs. Grice was also impressed by the Aristotelian idea that sensory modalities seem to have 'proper objects'. He doubted that the qualia theory can do justice to the fact that seeing is a way of finding out how things are by detecting such things as colors and shapes, whereas hearing is a matter of detecting sounds. And he doubted, moreover, that the qualia theory could explain why it is not possible to see sounds or hear colors. The proper-objects view locates the differentia of sensory modalities in their representational content, rather than in their qualitative character. Earlier in this chapter we considered some general reasons for being sympathetic with this idea: I argued that Peacocke's 'sensational properties' of experience are (in his sense) representational after all. This argument turned on enriching the account of what can be experienced (of the representational content of experience) so as to allow that we can see, for example, such things as the appearances of things. (I return to this theme in chapter 5.) In any event, it would seem that the proper-objects approach faces problems too: For example, it is frequently possible to perceive one and the same property or state of affairs by means of different senses.

The enactive approach allows us to incorporate elements from both the qualia and the proper objects view. What differentiates the senses, on the enactive approach, is that they are each modes of awareness, in the first instance, of different structured *appearance* spaces. Sight and touch are ways of encountering one and the same environment. But they differ in that, in each case, the encounter with the environment is an encounter with different patterns of appearance. Vision is a process of gleaning how things are, apart from how they appear, from the active exploration of structured looks space (e.g., the space of perspectival properties). Touch differs in being a mode of awareness of one and the same environment, but as mediated by patterns in how things *feel*. When we talk about the common content of visual, auditory, and tactile experiences, we are describing what is experienced in a way that abstracts away from how things appear (how they look, feel, sound, etc.).

Sensory modalities may in this way be individuated by means of their corresponding appearance structures (or objects). That is to say, we can endorse Aristotle's view that each of the senses has proper objects. The proper object of each sense is the type of appearance (looks, sounds, etc.) that is made available uniquely to that sense. Because the laws governing the relation between the environment and the several appearance spaces are different, there will be features of the environment (e.g., color) that are not available to all the senses. This is compatible with its being the case that the senses enable one, by means of one's encounter with appearances, to come into contact with how things are apart from how they appear.

We must not overdo the significance of the fact that it is in this way possible to individuate the senses by reference to their distinctive objects. For at the ground of our encounter with these different objects—appearances in one modality or another—is sensorimotor skill.

To appreciate this point, let's consider a particular example: that in visual experience we represent objects as given all at once, arrayed in a manifold. We experience, in this sense, a visual field. As Martin (1992) has noticed, this is a feature of what it is like to learn about the environment by seeing which does not hold for touch.[20] As Martin explains, in sight we experience "objects external to one as arranged in physical space" (1992, 210). Tactile experience, on the other hand, "is experience of objects as they come into contact with one's body; one is aware of one's body and its limits and so aware of objects coming into contact with one's body as they discernibly affect those limits. Normal visual experience is essentially experience of objects as they fall within the visual field; tactual experience is essentially experience of objects as they press from the outside onto the limits of a felt sensory field" (210). Martin notices that this "structural difference between the experiences" of sight and touch in part explains why the sense-datum theory has seemed so attractive in philosophical theories of sight, but not of touch. In the former case, sense data are brought on to explain the possibility of hallucination. Sense data are that of which we are aware when we are not really seeing what we think we see. But no such need arises in the case of touch. You are undergoing a tactile hallucination if your hand is restricted in movement in precisely the way it would be if it were pressed flat onto a wooden table, when in fact there is no wooden table there. There is no need to suppose that there is some kind of mental entity (a sense datum) that is preventing one's hand from moving to explain the hallucination.

Martin introduces these points in the service of skepticism about the prospects of accounting for the different varieties of perception (corresponding to the different modalities) under the rubric of a single, all-purpose theory. But his points actually serve to direct attention to just the materials needed for such a general theory.

Consider that to feel a table—to learn about it by touch—is to encounter it in such a way that one's movements are, in appropriate ways, impeded by the table. In general, one might say, to feel a shape or texture of a surface is, in this way, to allow one's movement to be molded by that which one touches. For something to feel this way or that (round, large, flat, rough, soft) is for it to condition the possibilities of movement of the palpating hand or body part in corresponding ways. The roundness, of course, exists apart from how it affects the probing hand. But for something to feel round (i.e., to appear round to the tactile sense) is precisely for it to affect the movement of the probing hand in a family of related ways. A sphere is such that if one moves one's hand in certain ways, one will have certain sensations. Tactile perception is a mode of awareness of the environment that is mediated by a particular network of sensorimotor patterns (by a set of ways our movements affect our sensory states).

The notion of sensorimotor dependence is of suitable generality to play a basic role in an account of the nature of sensory modalities. The idea, as we have considered throughout, is that how things look, smell, sound, or feel (etc.) depends, in complicated but systematic ways, on one's movement. The sensory modalities differ in the distinctive forms that this dependence takes. We have just considered features of the sensorimotor dependencies characteristic of touch. Sight has its own characteristic forms of sensorimotor dependence. As we have noticed, how things look varies in systematic ways as one moves one's eyes, head, or body relative to the environment. A simple illustration of this is the fact that as you move, objects come into and out of view. What Gibson calls the occluding edge of one object "wipes out" surface, while at its trailing edge surface is uncovered (Bruce and Green [1985] 1990). Importantly, this is reversible occlusion, and so is easily differentiated from the obliteration of things around one. This is an illustration of the manner in which perceptual exploration is structured by reliable patterns of sensorimotor dependence. A second example comes from patterns of "flow" in the optic field. Forward movement induces radial expansion in optic flow, while backward movement generates radial contraction. A distinct pattern of optic flow is generated by flight across the sky (as by a bird or a plane). The existence of such patterns in optic flow depends on the availability of distinctively visual patterns of sensorimotor contingency.

Note that there is an important relationship between invariant properties of the ambient optic array, discussed earlier, and regularities governing sensorimotor contingencies. So, for example, the invariance encountered as one walks around a rectangular table corresponds to a pattern of organization in the relevant sensorimotor contingencies.

On the view being developed here, then, the senses are modes of awareness of one and the same environment as mediated by different patterns of sensorimotor contingency. From the side of the object, what differentiates seeing and touching are their different objects (say, looks as opposed to feels). But from the side of the perceiver, what differentiates seeing from touching are the different patterns of activity in which seeing and touching respectively consist.

There is a superficial tension between the proposal that the sensory modalities can be individuated by the patterns of sensorimotor dependence governing them, and the proposal regarding the answer to Molyneux's question in section 3.8, that what enables touch and sight to share a common spatial content is that they *agree* in their sensorimotor structure. The key to resolving this apparent tension is to recognize that we need to be highly sensitive to considerations regarding the level at which sensorimotor isomorphism obtains (or fails to obtain). At a low level of characterization, the modalities are radically different, implicating distinct forms of sensorimotor pattern. It is possible to abstract from these differences, however, and it is when we do this that we can recognize the similarities between vision and TVSS (discussed later in this section), and also the common sensorimotor structures thanks to which vision and touch can both represent common spatial qualities.

On this account of the nature of sensory modalities, the senses are not merely channels by which information about the environment reaches the central nervous system, as argued recently by Keeley (2001). This view is too liberal in what it counts as a sense. On Keeley's view, for example, the vomeronasal system (which controls human and animal responses to pheromones and explains such facts as that the menstrual cycles of women living in a college dormitory tend to become synchronized, as found by McClintock [1971]) is a sensory modality. We can agree with Keeley that humans appear to be sensitive to vomeronasal variations. Such variations give rise to definite chemical and behavioral responses. Likewise, we may agree that vomeronasal sensitivity to pheromones constitutes an avenue whereby information about the environment reaches the central nervous system. But these facts are not sufficient to make it the case that we *perceive* vomeronasally. Consider, first, that there are no vomeronasal appearances, in the way that there are visual and tactile appearances. Vomeronasal information may make it more likely, for example, that an animal finds another physically attractive. But the animal does not find the other attractive *vomeronasally* (i.e., in a vomeronasal respect). Vomeronasal states may influence our feelings, attitudes, actions, and so forth, but they do not inform perceivers as to how things stand in the environment. To concede all this, however, and this is a second point, is to concede that there are no vomeronasal experiences. There is no activity of exploring how things are as mediated by one's encounter with how they vomeronasally appear.

Third, and as a consequence of the first two considerations, even animals in whom the vomeronasal system is highly effective do not master the patterns of vomeronasal motor contingencies that mediate their causal influence. That is, there is nothing analagous to knowing how to position one's nose to pick up a good scent, or the better to smell something, in the domain of vomeronasal information.[21]

The upshot of these points is that the vomeronasal system appears to be a channel whereby information from the environment reaches the central nervous system, which is not a sensory modality. Keeley's account of the senses may go astray because it fails to make allowance for the fact that perception is a mode of activity on the part of the whole animal. It cannot be represented in terms of merely passive, and internal, processes of the kind involved in vomeronasal sensitivity.

It is also important to appreciate that we cannot individuate perceptual modalities by physical or physiological criteria alone. This is demonstrated by consideration of sensory substitution systems such as Bach-y-Rita's tactile-visual substitution system (TVSS), mentioned above in section 3.8 and in chapter 1. TVSS is a mode of quasi-seeing without any involvement of eyes or visual cortex.

It is worth reminding ourselves of the details of the case. (For a recent, brief review, see Bach-y-Rita and Kercel 2002.) The subject is outfitted with a head-mounted camera that is wired up to electrodes (say, on the tongue) in such a way that visual information presented to the camera produces patterns of activation on the tongue. For subjects who are active (who control the information received by the camera by manipulations of themselves and the camera), it becomes possible, in a matter of hours, to make quasi-visual perceptual judgments. For example, subjects can report the number, size, spatial arrangement, and so forth of objects at a distance from themselves across the room. On the basis of this perception, they are enabled to reach out and grasp, to make swatting or grabbing movements of the hand. In addition, Bach-y-Rita reports that these subjects experience certain well-known visual illusions such as the waterfall illusion (Bach-y-Rita and Kercel 2002).

In what does the *visual* character, such as it is, of these perceptual experiences consist (O'Regan and Noë 2001a,b; Hurley and Noë 2003a and, especially, 2003b)? The preceeding discussion allows us to frame an account in two ways. First, we might notice that TVSS enables perception of *visual* qualities, that is, of looks. One can track perspectival visible features such as the way the apparent size changes as one moves with respect to the object. But second, this account in terms of the space of visual appearances is grounded on the more basic fact that the laws of sensorimotor contingency governing the quasi-vision of TVSS are like those of normal vision, at least to some substantial degree (e.g., at the appropriate level of abstraction).

Importantly, we cannot explain the quasi-visual character of experience with TVSS by appealing to the involvement of the eyes, or the visual cortex, for there is no involvement of eyes and visual cortex.[22] TVSS depends on the camera's tactile stimulation of the body resulting in activity in somatosensory (tactile) cortex.

One could object that the notions of *eye* and *visual cortex* are functional ones. For adapted subjects, the camera and the temporal cortex (which is the anatomical region that instantiates somatosensory cortex in normal subjects) *become* eye and visual cortex.

This is exactly right, but it amounts to no objection at all. What makes an eye an *eye* is its deployment in the context of a network of sensorimotor contigencies. What makes a locus of brain activity a locus of *visual* activity is, precisely, the fact that this activity is deployed in the services of this larger sensorimotor task (Hurley and Noë 2003a,b). The implications of this need to be stressed, however: What makes eye- and visual cortex–dependent perceptual activity *visual* are not the intrinsic qualities of the patterns of stimulation and activation they set up, but rather the overarching sensorimotor dependencies, and knowledge thereof, that govern this neural activity.

Perceptual modalities, we have seen, are autonomous of the physical systems (the organs) in which they are embodied. To understand the nature of vision, as distinct from touch or hearing, you must focus on the differences in the respective patterns of sensorimotor dependence. Nevertheless, it turns out that there is good reason to believe that the sensorimotor dependencies are themselves determined by low-level details of the physical systems on which our sensory systems depend. The eye and the visual parts of the brain form a most subtle instrument indeed, and thanks to this instrument, sensory stimulation varies in response to movement in precise ways. To see *as we do*, you must then have a sensory organ and a body like ours.

This raises the worry about sensorimotor chauvinism (raised by Clark and Toribio 2001; Clark 2002) considered briefly at the end of chapter 1. I am in a better position now to develop the reply I made then: Granted, the enactive view is chauvinistic, but only to an acceptable degree. In virtue of *what* can the visual systems of the human, the crab, and the bumblebee all be deemed *visual* systems? Is it because they all give rise to the same kind of experiences, qualitatively speaking? How far must we commit to accepting that? According to the enactive view, there is sufficient high-level, gross sensorimotor isomorphism between these different perceptual systems to count one and all as *visual* systems. There are also very many low-level sensorimotor differences, and these differences are sufficient to make the visual "experience" of the bee and the person different. But isn't this just the consequence we want?

Sensory modalities are *ways* of exploring the environment drawing on sensorimotor knowledge (O'Regan and Noë 2001a). The qualia theory was right to insist that there are qualitative differences among the modalities. But these qualitative differences are differences precisely in the ways how things appear informs us of how things are, differences available to us by way of our knowledge of sensorimotor dependencies. We have already considered that the proper objects view is also right: The modalities differ in which appearances matter.

3.11   Sensation and Perception

Nicholas Humphrey (1992, 78–81) offers a different interpretation of tactile vision (what he calls "skin vision"). According to Humphrey, although tactile vision may be a form of visual *perception*, it is accompanied by tactile *sensation*. Block (2003) develops a similar idea in a recent critical comment on a paper of mine and Susan Hurley's. Block writes: "Hurley and Noë appear to presuppose that visual phenomenology [of TVSS] is shown by the *spatial* function of TVSS—e.g. that tactile 'size' increases as you approach. But non-visual senses might be spatial in the same way, e.g. bat sonar . . . Perhaps TVSS is a case of spatial perception via tactile sensation (maybe Braille is too)" (2003, 286).

In support of this claim, Humphrey and Block both call attention to the fact that, for example, Bach-y-Rita (1996, 50) himself admits that "even during task performance with the sensory system, the subject can perceive purely tactile sensations when asked to concentrate on these sensations."

The fact that one can direct one's attention to tactile sensations accompanying TVSS *does not* show that the qualitative content of TVSS is tactile. For one thing, it doesn't show that those accompanying sensations are themselves part of the perceptual experience.

This is perhaps clearer in a different kind of example. In order to perceive with a cane, the blind person must have feeling in the hand. But to feel the world with a cane is not a way of touching with or in the hand. (If the feeling is anywhere, it is at the end of the cane, where one has *no* sensations.) As O'Shaughnessy (2000) has observed, the sensations in the hand that enable you to perceive with a cane are *outside* the scope of perceptual attention and so, for this reason, are not part of the perceptual experience itself. Indeed, precisely this point can be made about normal perception by means of the hand. When you feel the shape of a bottle you may have sensations (e.g., as of the bottle's coolness), but the sensations of coolness are not part of your experience of the bottle's shape. Indeed, as O'Shaughnessy notes (mentioned in chapter 1), you could feel the bottle's shape even if your hands were numb.

When you do attend to the sensations that accompany perceptual experience, you turn your attention away from the experience. You may attend to muscular strain in the eyes as you move and squint, or to the weight of the glasses on your nose, but this doesn't show that those sensations are *visual*, or that *visual* experience has kinesthetic phenomenology.

Humphrey and Block seem to make two questionable claims. First, they hold that sensation and perception can be completely dissociated. For example, Block writes: "One intriguing possibility is that there may be an independent phenomenology both to sensation (grounded in brain state) and to perception (grounded in the function of that brain state). Who knows—maybe *both* traditional functionalism and physicalism will turn out to be partially true!" (2003, 286). This possibility of dissociation is an important principle in Humphrey's theory of consciousness. According to Humphrey (1992), sensation and perception constitute two separate and autonomous channels; sensation developed in evolutionary time first, as a capacity for animals to keep track of what is happening to them, in and on their bodies. He gives "skin vision" as an example of the dissociation of visual perception and visual sensation. He also cites Kohler's work on inverting spectacles as further evidence of the dissociation of sensation and perception. Perceptual adaptation to inverting goggles, he argues, does not involve any change in the character of one's sensation (as has been argued by Harris).

Second, Humphrey and Block seem to assume that perceptual phenomenology is determined by the character of the accompanying sensations. Humphrey writes: "The phenomenology of sensory experiences came first. Before there were any other kinds of phenomena there were "raw sensations"—tastes, smells, tickles, pains, sensations of warmth, of light, of sound, and so on" (1992, 42).

One reason for doubting this second assumption, as we have seen, is the fact that sensational accompaniments of perception are not in general constituents of perceptual experience. But there is a stronger reason as well. Let us grant that TVSS is qualitatively distinct from vision and that the phenomenology of TVSS is not visual. Notice, however, that TVSS is also qualitatively distinct from touch. TVSS-experience presents the world in a way that is quite definitely not the way the world is presented in normal touch. This comes out, for example, in the fact that TVSS allows for experiences of a spatial manifold (as discussed earlier). Even if it is the case that TVSS is accompanied by tactile sensations, it is clear that those tactile sensations do not suffice to determine the modal quality of the corresponding experience. At best, it would seem, the character of the accompanying sensations makes a contribution to the overall phenomenology of perception.

What determines the modal quality of TVSS? The enactive approach offers an explanation. The enactive approach accounts for the respects in which TVSS and normal vision are alike, and also the respects in which they are unalike. They are similar to the extent that there is a sensorimotor isomophism between them. At higher levels—concerning, for example, the effects of gross movements—there is a strong sensorimotor isomorphism. Movements of the head and body relative to objects produce similar patterns of sensory change. The laws of sensorimotor contingency that must be mastered by the perceiver in both cases are similar or identical. At lower levels, of course, substantial differences exist. It is plausible that only an electrode array of the same degree of complexity and refinement as the retina could support just the same visual sensorimotor laws. Moreover, the nature of the camera-electrode system is so different from that of the eyes-brain system that there must be tremendous low-level sensorimotor differences;

that is, the effects of movement on low-level details of sensory stimulation is enormously different in the two cases.

The upshot of this discussion of TVSS is that we can accept Block's and Humphrey's claims about the dissociability of sensation and perception, but only if we also recognize that their second claim—that sensations determine phenomenology—is false. It is necessary to distinguish sensations that may (or may not) accompany perception in a modality from the features of an experience thanks to which it is qualitatively visual, tactile, or of some other modality.

One way to bring out what is wrong with Humphrey's theory of sensations—and indeed, with the whole empiricist approach to perception associated with Thomas Reid—is that it fails to do justice to the intentionality of perceptual experience—that is, to the fact that experience always presents the world as being some way to one. This issue comes to the fore, for example, in Humphrey's discussion of inverting goggles. He writes:

Suppose you were to wear special "up-down inverting spectacles" in front of your eyes, so that even while you yourself remained upright your retinal image were to be permanently turned the wrong way up. In this situation the perceptual mechanism would make no allowance for the transformation of the image, and so—initially at least—you would see both the image to be the wrong way up (which it is) and the external world to be the wrong way up (which it is not). Hence you would be bound to make perceptual mistakes—pointing up for an object when you should point down, calling "top" "bottom," and so on. (Humphrey 1992, 76)

When Humphrey says that you see the image to be the wrong way up, he means (as he makes clear in this passage) that "if you attend to visual sensation it will be apparent that the image at your retina has now turned around: parts of the image that previously appeared nearer the top of your eye socket are now nearer the bottom, parts that were nearer the right side are now nearer the left, and so on" (1992, 76).

But this is mistaken. It just isn't the case that it is apparent to one that the retinal image is turned around. The retinal image doesn't enter into your experience at all! Rather, when you wear the goggles, spatial relations in the visible environment *look* different; it looks as if what is up is down, and so on. The goggles produce these changes in your experience, but these are not changes in the character of your sensations; they are changes in how the experience perceptually presents things as being. We are in the domain of perception here, not sensation. Insofar as sensation ought to figure in an account of perception, it is sensation not in the sense of "raw feeling," but rather in the sense of appearances. But then sensation enters into experience as part of the way the experience presents the world as being. Sensations, in this sense, belong to the intentional content of the experience.

The enactive view, as I have urged earlier, does offer an explanation of the spatial content of perceptual experience, and so of *intramodal* differences in experience.

3.12 A Note on Sensorimotor Knowledge

I have been arguing that vision depends on sensorimotor knowledge (O'Regan and Noë 2001a). It is this knowledge of the way sensory stimulation varies as a function of movement that is the basis of our ability to have world-presenting sensory experience. In this chapter I have claimed that perceptual experience, in whatever modality, acquires spatial content thanks to the perceiver's knowledge of the way sensory stimulation depends on movement. In chapter 2 I argued that the ground of our sense of perceptual presence (of, e.g., environmental detail, occluded surfaces, colors, etc.) is not only the fact that we stand in definite sensorimotor relations to the features in question, but that we know that we do.

Throughout I have taken pains to emphasize that the knowledge in question is practical, not propositional. The relevant sensorimotor knowledge consists in the possession of practical abilities. One reason why I refer to this complex of abilities as constituting *knowledge* is in order to call attention to the foundational role these abilities play with respect to genuinely knowledge-involving cognitive capacities. For example, as I argue in chapter 6, observational concepts are concepts whose understanding is constituted, in part, by sensorimotor skills. This is a theme that has already begun to emerge in the discussion in this chapter. When you experience something as cubical, you experience it as presenting a definite sensorimotor profile. That is, you experience it as something whose appearance would vary in precise ways as you move in relation to it, or as it moves in relation to you. You have an implicit practical mastery of these patterns of change. It is this implicit practical mastery in which, for the most part, your eventual appreciation of the observational concept *cubical* consists.

A second reason to refer to sensorimotor skills as constituting a kind of knowledge is that, as touched on in chapter 2, there is no sharp line where your perceptual awareness of something stops and your mere *thought* awareness of it starts. I can think of the Eiffel Tower right now, but not perceive it. (It's in Paris. I'm in Berkeley.) But I am visually aware, in that special sense I tried to explain in chapter 2, of occluded portions of the scene around me, even though they are, strictly speaking, out of view. By calling sensorimotor skill "knowledge," I am signaling the that we should be open to the possibility that thought and experience are, in important ways, continuous.

Crucially, sensorimotor knowledge is not propositional. In particular, it is not knowledge of propositions describing the sensory effects of possible or actual movements. There are, in fact, decisive objections to the idea that perception and perceptual experience could be grounded on that sort of propositional knowledge. First, it is unlikely that perceivers (human and otherwise) actually have that knowledge. One might wonder whether it would be possible, even in principle, to state, in propositional terms, what it is that a perceiver knows in virtue of which he or she is able to have world-presenting perceptual experiences. Whether or not this is so, from the fact that a person has a certain ability (e.g., to dance), it hardly follows that she has knowledge of the propositions that would describe that ability.

Second, propositional knowledge of counterfactuals along the lines of "if you move like this, your experience will change like this" could not be the basis of the grasp of spatial content, because the counterfactuals themselves presuppose a prior grasp on such content. The idea here is that it is *because* we experience the tomato as three-dimensional and voluminous that we are committed to the relevant counterfactual conditionals.[23] To suppose otherwise would be to make the behaviorist error of supposing that effects are logical constructions of their causes (Putnam 1963). This criticism may lose some of its punch when we acknowledge that there is in fact no satisfactory *alternative* theory of perceptual experience of spatial content. The standard view in vision science would be that we should explain how the brain builds up a 3-D representation of an object, and then appeal to this representation as the ground of perceivers' knowledge of the infinity of counterfactuals describing the effects of movement on sensation.[24] The problem with this sort of approach, however, is that it promises more than it can deliver. We may have some idea of how the visual system could build up a detailed spatial representation of an object (drawing on work in the computational theory of vision). But we have no satisfactory account whatsoever of how the existence of such a representation is supposed to enable us to *experience* objects in space. How could the existence of an internal representation explain my sense of the presence to vision of a part of the object that I am unable to see directly?

It is also unclear whether there would be need to suppose that perceivers possess propositional *knowledge* of the relevant counterfactuals, as opposed to, say, belief.[25] The work of the enactive approach is done by perceivers' *expectations* of the sensory effects of movement, not their knowledge of those effects. After all, the stage tomato will look solidly 3-D if, in looking at it, the perceiver takes it as presenting a 3-D sensorimotor profile, whether or not it does.

Because the enactive approach is not committed to a propositional account of sensorimotor skill, it is immune to the problems such an approach would face. Nevertheless, we still need a fuller account of the nature of sensorimotor skills. Until we can provide such an account, there may be legitimate grounds for worry that, for sensorimotor skills to do explanatory work, their possession will have to amount to the possession of knowledge of the relevant counterfactuals. Recall, the cube presents itself to me *as* a cube, precisely because I understand, implicitly, that its appearance would change in determinate ways were I to move in respect of it (or were it to move in respect of me). What content can be given to the claim that this sensorimotor ability is *not* propositional knowledge?

To reply to this worry it is not enough to argue—in the manner of some linguists—that the knowledge in question is *tacit*. Tacitness would explain why it is that perceivers are unable to say what it is they know when they know how to see, but it wouldn't address the deeper explanatory worry. According to the enactive approach, perceptual content becomes available to experience when perceivers have practical mastery of the ways sensory stimulation varies as a result of movement. It would be unsatisfying to explain this mastery by appeal to the perceiver's tacit grasp of propositions describing the sensory effects of movement. First, one can reasonably ask: How could knowing that enable us to *experience* anything? Second, as discussed earlier, this seems to put the cart before the horse; knowledge of the propositions (tacit or otherwise) is (as Peacocke has put it, in conversation) *consequent* on the experience.

The solution, I think, is to insist that the mastery in question be purely practical and not a matter of the knowledge of propositions (tacit or otherwise). Instead of comparing perceiving to speech, we should instead compare it to gestural devices of communication. Gesture plays an important role in communication, but perceivers rarely know what gestures they make and when. If you ask someone to report what she said during a conversation, she is likely to be able to comply. But she is much less likely to be able to describe the gestures she made. Gesture knowledge is body knowledge; it belongs to our pre-intellectual habits, skills, anticipations, forms of readiness. Even if, as a matter of fact, complex abilities—like the ability to dance—are amenable to characterization by propositions, it would not follow that being able to dance consists in knowing those propositions. There is no sense, then, in which the enactive approach is committed to the idea that perceivers have cognitive access to the content of experience prior to their grasp of sensorimotor knowledge. Sensorimotor knowledge is basic.

This is obviously a delicate issue about which much more needs to be said. I want to conclude by commenting on Stanley and Williamson's recent attack (2001) on the legitimacy of the distinction between practical and propositional knowledge. This challenge might seem to threaten the enactive approach by depriving it of a needed conception of practical knowledge of sensorimotor dependencies.

Stanley and Williamson argue, rather in the spirit of ordinary language philosophy, that it is a mistake to think of know-how as consisting of abilities. They deny that, generally speaking, from the fact that someone knows how to ϕ it follows that he or she *can* ϕ. A ski instructor might know how to perform a certain tricky jump, without being able to perform it herself, just as a pianist might know how to play a piece, even though he can't, because he's just lost his arms in an accident. I don't share Stanley and Williamson's robust intuitions here. I would have thought that if a ski instructor can't do the jump, then she doesn't know how to do it either, even if she might be able to teach someone else how to do it. What she knows is how to teach someone to do it, not how to do it. She knows how the jump is done, but not how to do it. Sadly, the same is true of the pianist. He may retain all sorts of cognate knowledge—relevant to the description, critical evaluation, or teaching of how to play a piece of music—but when he lost his arms, he lost his know-how. For the knowledge was, precisely, arm-dependent. Stanley and Williamson also point out that being able to do something is no guarantee that you know how to do it. After all, they say, you can win the lottery, even if you don't know how to win the lottery. Maybe, but I would be inclined to say that anyone who can win a lottery does know how to win it. Knowing how to win a lottery is knowing how to enter into it fairly.

Stanley and Williamson are on somewhat firmer ground, I think, when they argue that knowing-how does in fact consist of knowing that certain propositions are true. They reason that when you know how to ride a bicycle, say, what you know is that some particular activity is the way to ride a bicycle, and you know that, as they put it, under the 'practical mode of presentation'. It is possible to know the proposition that such and such is the way to ride a bicycle without knowing it under the practical mode of presentation. In that case, you know that something is the way to ride a bike without knowing how to ride a bike yourself. In a similar way, John can know that that man's pants are on fire, without realizing that he is that man (say, because he doesn't realize he's looking in a mirror). In a case like this John knows the proposition that his pants are on fire, but not under the first-personal mode of presentation.

I said that Stanley and Williamson are on firmer ground when they argue that knowledge-how is knowledge-that. In good measure this is because their attack on the distinction is merely technical. Let us grant their claim that all knowledge-how is knowledge-that. Crucially, knowledge-how is a special kind of knowledge-that. The familiar distinction is preserved, only relocated as a distinction between different ways of grasping or understanding propositions. If they are right, then, if sensorimotor knowledge is practical knowledge, it is knowledge of propositions describing the effects of movement grasped under the practical mode of presentation.

We have considered reasons to doubt that there are any propositions that might play the role of that which is known (under the practical mode of presentation or any other) when one knows how to perceive. If this is right, then we may find ourselves with strong theoretical grounds for thinking that sensorimotor knowledge is nonpropositional know-how, a conclusion incompatible with Stanley and Williamson's analysis.

Whatever we say about this, the enactive approach requires the availability of a conception of practical knowledge, and Stanley and Willamson's considerations do not, as far as I can tell, do anything to make such a conception unavailable.

4 Colors Enacted

A color has many faces.
—Josef Albers

4.1 The Problem of Color

When you visually experience a plate as circular, you do so relying on your implicit knowledge of the way the plate's appearance—its look—varies as your relation to the plate changes. You encounter its real shape (its circularity) in your experience, thanks to your encounters with its merely apparent shape (its elliptical look). The apparent shape—the perspectival shape—is a genuine property of the scene, but it is a property whose nature is fixed by the relation between the object and the conditions in which it is viewed. When you see how a thing looks from here (e.g., elliptical), you find out something about how things are (e.g., circular), and you find out something about how things are *around you*. To experience something as *elliptical from here* is to experience it as occupying a certain place in your sensorimotor space, for example, as being such as to be blocked from view by *this* sort of an occluder, or as being something whose outline could be traced by such and such a movement, and so forth. To experience it as circular, despite its looking elliptical, is to understand the way its appearance would change, if the conditions in which you view it were to change (e.g., if your spatial relation to it were to change).

Can we extend this sort of enactive, sensorimotor account to the experience of color? There is an influential line of thought about color experience, which I call *the qualia theory* (following Pettit 2003a), that answers this question negatively. According to the qualia theory, to experience something as looking red, say, is to have a certain kind of experience. The experienced quality of redness, in this view, is a property of the experience—a sensational property or quale—one that (partly) fixes what it is like to have the experience, and one that is immediately revealed or overt in the experience (Johnston 1992; Pettit 2003a). From the standpoint of the qualia theory, two individuals who are identical in all behavioral dispositions (including their sensorimotor skills and discriminatory capacities) could differ in what it is like for them to experience something red looking. This is the hypothesis of the inverted spectrum (see, e.g., Shoemaker 1982; Palmer 1999b). Furthermore, from the standpoint of the qualia theory, a person could have normal color-pertinent sensorimotor skills but lack color experience altogether. This is the so-called zombie argument (see, e.g., Chalmers 1996).

The qualia theory is a theory of color experience. It is not a theory of color, not a theory of what colors are. For this reason, the qualia theory is compatible with a range of different accounts of the metaphysics of color. Physicalists, who hold that colors are physical properties of, for example, surfaces, and eliminativists, who deny that anything is colored (colors, on such a view, are merely subjective "effects" in perceivers), can both accept the qualia theory as an analysis of what it is like to *experience* colors (say, of what it is for something to look red to one).

However metaphysically nonpartisan, the qualia theory is *not* compatible with an enactive account of color experience. For the qualia theory analyzes what it is for something to look a particular way to one with respect to color in a way that is independent of the sorts of skills that are basic on the enactive account.

My aim in this chapter is to present an enactive account of color experience. The first task is to make the case for such an account, and this depends on exhibiting the *sensorimotor profile* of color. The enactive account is not metaphysically nonpartisan however; it suggests an account of the nature of color. My second task in this chapter is to develop such an account and explain its relation to other theories of color. I challenge the qualia theory on its home field, so to speak. I argue that the qualia theory is weakest where it is supposedly strongest, namely, in the account it provides of the phenomenology of color experience.

4.2   Colors Have Rich Sensorimotor Profiles

How a thing looks with respect to color varies as it moves in relation to a light source. If you rotate a tomato, the part of the tomato facing the light will look brighter than the part facing away from it. If you now move the tomato away, say, from a household light (e.g., a tungsten bulb), which contains a large amount of long wavelength light, into the daylight coming in through the window, which contains equal portions of light at different wavelengths across the spectrum, you will notice changes in the way the tomato looks with respect to color.

In general, changes in ambient light produce changes in the appearance of colored objects. The apparent color of a car in the fluorescent light of the garage is strikingly different from its apparent color in bright daylight. As clouds move to block the sun, and as the day progresses, the car perceptibly changes its color appearance. The way a thing looks with respect to color depends on the character of the illuminating light, and it varies as the character of lighting changes.

The apparent color of an object also varies as the *perceiver* moves in relation to the object, even when the conditions of illumination, and when the object's position relative to a light source, do not change. For example, the specular highlights on the surface of a clean, new automobile vary as viewing geometry varies. Specular highlights are frequently the color of the incident light itself, reflecting white in the sunshine, and also the colors of, for example, street lights. As you move in relation to the car, or as it moves in relation to you, the apparent color of the car's surface may visibly change.

The way a thing looks with respect to hue and brightness depends not only on viewing geometry and lighting, but also on the chromatic properties of surrounding and contrasting objects. The white ceilings of a house surrounded by lawns may appear bright green on a sunny day (Albers 1963, 45). A card may look white when placed against a dark background, only to reveal itself to be gray or even black when moved to a lighter background.[1] Josef Albers gives numerous examples of this sort of simultaneous color contrast. For example, if you take a single strip of ochre paper and cut it in two, placing one piece on dark blue paper and the other on bright yellow paper, the two pieces of ochre paper will look strikingly different.

The strip against blue paper will appear much lighter than the one against yellow paper (Albers 1963, 77). In another paper construction, Albers makes a cross out of grayish paper and places it on a yellow background, where it looks decidedly violet. Against a violet background, however, the same piece of paper looks yellowish and lighter. In these sorts of ways, as Albers writes, colors act on each other by "pulling" or "pushing" "each other into different appearances (toward both greater difference and greater similarity)" (Albers 1963, 33).

A very familiar example of simultaneous contrast effects is provided by television. TV produces images by emitting light. To create darkness—for example, the black of someone's leather coat, or of a cave, say—TV can only *fail* to emit light. When a TV is off (i.e., when it fails to emit any light), its screen typically looks gray or sometimes greenish gray. In this condition, it fails to emit light altogether. But the black of the leather jacket in a show does not look greenish gray; it looks black. How can the TV give rise to an image that is perceptibly darker than the entirely non-light-emitting screen? This effect is produced by the presence of contrasting lights.

John Ruskin offers a telling illustration of this sort of "push-pull" effect in the domain of color. His subject is the technical art of painting. He writes:

When grass is lighted strongly by the sun in certain directions, it is turned from green into a peculiar and somewhat dusty-looking yellow. If we had been born blind, and were suddenly endowed with sight on a piece of grass thus lighted in some parts by the sun, it would appear to us that part of the grass was green, and part a dusty yellow (very nearly of the colour of primroses); and if there were primroses near, we should think that the sunlighted grass was another mass of plants of the same sulphur-yellow colour. We should try to gather some of them, and then find that the colour went away from the grass when we stood between it and the sun, but not from the primroses; and by a series of experiments we should find out that the sun was really the cause of the colour in the one,—not in the other. We go through such processes of experiment unconsciously in childhood; and having come to conclusions touching the signification of certain colours, we always suppose that we *see* what we only know, and have hardly any consciousness of the real aspect of the signs we have learned to interpret. Very few people have any idea that sunlighted grass is yellow. (Ruskin [1856] 1971, 27)

According to Ruskin, the process of learning to perceive color is, precisely, a process of coming to understand the behavior of color as we move and as environmental conditions change (i.e., "by a series of experiments"). This learning takes place "unconsciously in childhood" and later prevents us (we would-be painters) from noticing, for example, the effects of sunlight on grass. Of course, the point is that once someone calls to our attention the fact that the green grass does not look green when it is lighted by the sun, we immediately recognize that this is right.

Perceivers are in general implicitly familiar with the way apparent color varies as we move with respect to what we look at, or as other *color-critical* conditions change, (e.g., changes in the character of ambient light, or in the colors of contrasting objects, etc.). Perceivers implicitly understand the patterns governing this sort of variation, just as they implicitly understand the way that the apparent shape of an object changes as they move in relation to the object.

The phenomenon of *color constancy* demonstrates that perceivers possess this sort of implicit knowledge. We have noticed, for example, the way in which the color of the car may change as lighting conditions vary. Despite these changes in apparent color, and despite specular colors, perceivers are usually able to recognize, say, that the car is a uniform and unchanging red. (Broackes 1992 gives this example.) We see the uniformity despite, or behind or beneath (as it were), the variable appearance. We do not confuse changes in the apparent color as color-critical conditions change with changes in the underlying actual color. For example, suppose you enter a room and see that the wall is a uniform shade of white. You also see that the wall is brighter here, where it falls in direct sunlight, than it is there, where it falls in shadow. Differences in brightness, however, mean differences in color. You see the uniformity of color despite the evident nonuniformity of different parts of the wall's surface. Crucially, the changes or nonuniformities in illumination *do* affect the apparent color of the object—after all, they affect the brightness and perceived hue of the surface—but they do not affect our experience of the *actual* color. As perceivers we are familiar with the way the apparent color of a thing changes as its relation to the surrounding light, or our relation to the surrounding light changes. We experience color as that which is, in a wide range of cases, *invariant* amid that apparent variation.

In this way, then, color perception and shape perception are on a par. You experience the roundness of the plate in the fact that it looks elliptical from here and that its elliptical appearance changes (or would change) in precise ways as your relation to the plate, or the plate's relation to the environment, changes. In exactly this way, we experience the color of the wall in the fact that the apparent color of the wall varies as lighting changes. We are able to experience the actual color of the object as, so to speak, that condition which governs or regulates the way these changes unfold. We see the color of the wall in the way its appearance changes (in the way it interacts with the surrounding environment).

The analogy between the perception of color and the perception of shape may be extended. Just as it is not possible to see every aspect of an object from a single vantage point, so it is not possible to experience every aspect of an object's color all at once, from a single vantage point (as it were). The color of the object is no more completely visible under a single set of viewing conditions than is the shape of an object visible from a single vantage point. (Nor is it less visible.) How the thing looks with respect to color in these conditions is not enough to tell its color. In the same way, we can say that the shape of the object—say, its roundness—isn't visible from here.

The phenomenon of color constancy is a striking example of the phenomenon "presence in absence" described in chapter 2. Consider that although we can perceive a wall that is illuminated unevenly as uniform in color, it is also the case that when a wall is in this way illuminated unevenly, it is also visibly different with respect to color across its surface. For example, to match the color of different parts of the wall, you would need different color chips. Standard ways of characterizing color constancy as a phenomenon have a tendency to explain away the fact that we experience the wall as uniform in color even when we experience the surface as visibly differentiated with respect to color across its surface. The problem of color constancy, then, is better framed as a problem about perceptual presence. We experience the presence of a uniform color that, strictly speaking, we do not see. Or rather, the actual uniform color of the wall's surface is present in perception *amodally;* it is present but absent, in the same way as the *tomato's* backside, or the blocked parts of the cat.

Peacocke (1983) used color constancy to illustrate the difference between the *representational content* of an experience (how the world is represented by the experience) and the *qualitative* or *sensational properties* of experience (what the experience is like apart from its representational features). The experience of the wall here and there are the same in their representational content, but they differ nonrepresentationally in their qualitative character. This seems wrong: Just as our experience can present the circularity of the plate, even though the plate looks elliptical from here, so the experience can present the uniform color of the wall, even though the surface looks irregular in color. Crucially, we can experience the wall as uniform in color *and* as differently colored across its surface. Just as we can see that the plate looks circular *and* elliptical, so we can see the color is uniform *and* variable. Just as we see the circularity in the elliptical appearance, so we see the invariant color *in* the apparent variability. The color of the wall is present in absence; it is implicitly present.[2]

Our ability to perceive the wall's color depends on our implicit understanding of the ways its apparent color varies as color-critical conditions vary. At ground, our grasp of these dependencies is a kind of sensorimotor knowledge. We can distinguish two different kinds of sensorimotor dependencies.[3] (This distinction was first introduced in section 2.5.) Crucially, the perceptual experience of color depends on the perceiver's knowledge of *both* kinds of sensorimotor patterns.

Movement-dependent sensorimotor contingencies are patterns of dependence between sensory stimulation, on the one hand, and movements of the body, on the other. The way sensory stimulation is affected by changes in a perceiver's geometrical relation to an object is an example of this sort of movement-dependent sensorimotor pattern, as is the way stimulation varies as a result of the perceiver's manipulation of an object (e.g., turning it in relation to a light source). Consider two further examples of movement-dependent sensorimotor contingencies.

When you fixate a colored surface, the long, medium, and short wavelength-sensitive cones in the foveal region of your eye will respond in a manner determined by the spectral composition of the light reflected from the surface. Moving your eyes to the right, say, away from the surface, stimulates parafoveal receptors (where there are many more rods and fewer wavelength-sensitive cones). The characteristic change in stimulation as you move your eyes partly determines what it is like to look at something with that characteristic color. (This example is discussed in O'Regan and Noë 2001a.)

A second example turns on the fact that there is a yellow pigment in the fovea of the eye (called the macular pigment or the *macula lutea*). This pigment absorbs greater amounts of short wavelength light entering the eye than light of longer wavelengths. (See O'Regan and Noë 2001a and J. J. Clark 2002 for discussions of this.) As a result, the sensory effects of eye movements across blue, green, and red objects (i.e., across objects disposed to reflect relatively large amounts of short, medium, and long wavelength light, respectively) are strikingly different. The spectrum of light is "yellowed" when it falls on the central retina, and this effect is stronger for blues than it is for reds (Clark 2002).

These movement-dependent sensorimotor contingencies are complicated, and they are subpersonal (i.e., they hold independently of our conscious awareness, control, or effort). They are almost certainly partly constitutive of what it is like to experience the color of the surface. The distinction between personal and subpersonal is not very important in this domain. We control the movements of our bodies, and movements of our bodies produce sensory affects in the large and in the small. Think of the eye/brain as a sort of visual hand. Just as movements of the hand over an object produce sensory effects that depend, among other things, on the way the hand is built, so movements of the eye/brain produce sensory effects that depend on the way the eye/brain is built. Just as the neural (sensory) effects of probing an object with the hand vary depending on the shape of the object, so probing the surface with the eye/brain depends on the character of the object's surface, on such facts as its surface reflectance. The experience of color depends on such facts as that the object controls, at multiple levels, patterns of sensorimotor dependence (O'Regan and Noë 2001a).

Movement-dependent sensorimotor contingencies can be contrasted with *object-dependent* (or *environmental*, what J. J. Clark 2002 calls "ecological") sensorimotor contingencies. These are patterns of dependence between sensory stimulation and *the object's* movement, or the object's changing relation to its surrounding. Many of the sensorimotor patterns we have considered so far are environmental in this sense; that is, they are regularities determined by the relation between colored objects and the ambient light, the colors of surrounding objects, and so forth. Consider an additional example of an environmental principle of sensorimotor dependence. We are genuinely able to distinguish color *as an effect of illumination* and color *as an effect of object surface*. So, for example, we can usually see the difference between a room with green walls in natural lighting and a room whose white walls are bathed in green light. Langer and Gilchrist (2000) have demonstrated that in a simple scene of one reflectance (such as the one described), perceivers are able to disentangle color appearance as determined by *direct* illumination and color appearance as determined by *indirect* illumination, that is, by the illumination of surfaces by light reflected off the other surfaces (inter-reflections). The spectral composition of light is affected by the reflective properties of the surfaces (e.g., by the paint); therefore, to determine the color of the paint, one needs to compare the way the apparent color changes in, say, shadowed and unshadowed regions—that is, in regions where there is less or more direct light. The brightest regions (i.e., the regions with most direct light) will more strongly indicate the color of the illumination. The darkest regions, in contrast, where there is less direct illumination, will more strongly reflect the reflectance properties of the paint itself. Langer and Gilchrist's proposal suggests that sensitivity to the color of the walls as distinct from the color of the ambient light is something we can do because we are sensitive to the way *how things look* varies as a function of relations holding among surfaces, illumination, and environmental clutter (which is responsible for shadows).

In a case such as this, perceivers exercise implicit grasp not of the sensory effects of their own movement, but of the differential sensory effects of environmental relationships. Of course, there is a different strategy for discovering whether the apparent color of the room is determined by the illumination rather than the walls. Enter the room and pay attention to what happens to your skin! If your skin changes color when you enter, that's evidence that the controlling influence on color is the illumination. By testing *movement-dependent* sensorimotor contingencies in this way, you can determine color properties.

In chapter 3 I introduced (following Koenderink 1984b) the notion of the visual potential (with respect to shape) of a cube: This is the way its aspect changes as a result of movement (of the cube itself, or of the perceiver around the cube). Any movement determines a set of changes in perceived aspect; any set of changes in perceived aspects determines equivalence classes of possible movements. In the same way, then, we can speak of the visual potential of an object with respect to color. The way in which color appearance transforms as conditions change, however, is *much* more complicated. Movements of the perceiver or object relative to each other or relative to the light source, variations in the character of illuminating light, and variations in the colors of background or contrasting objects are all dimensions along which colors vary. However complicated, each color can be thought of as corresponding to a unique *color aspect profile*, a unique range of ways its color aspect transforms as the relevant kinds of movements (color-critical changes) occur.

To see the color of an object—to experience which color it has—is to discover its visual potential or color aspect profile; it is to grasp how its appearance changes or would change as color-critical conditions change. To experience something as red, then, is to experience not merely how it looks here and now, but how it would look as color-critical conditions vary. Only a perceiver with an understanding of these laws of transformation—who grasps the color aspect profile—can experience a determinate color. To experience a color you must grasp its color aspect profile, that is, its sensorimotor profile.

This is illustrated by a familiar phenomenon. To paint a wall the same color as an existing wall, it is not enough that you find paint that appears to match the color of the wall, namely, that matches it here and now. Perfect agreement between two patches here and now (under these conditions) doesn't guarantee agreement in color, for as conditions change, the actual differences in color between the patches may become apparent. To get a match, you need to investigate the ways the color changes over time as conditions vary. Sameness of color is a matter of potential appearance over time.

4.3   Looks Red

One might grant that our ability to experience something as having a determinate color depends on our practical grasp of the way its apparent color changes as conditions change, and that our possession of that knowledge is a condition of our having experience with that sort of content. But what is it to experience the apparent color? What is it for a car, say, to *look* red from here, in these viewing conditions? We know what it is for a plate to look elliptical from here. It is for it, say, to be such as would be perfectly occluded by an elliptical patch on the plane of occlusion. In what does the red look of a car (from here, under these circumstances) consist? How does a thing look when it looks red (as Pettit 2003a has asked)?

What makes this question difficult to answer is the *dis*analogy, ignored until now, between experiencing shapes and experiencing colors. When you see that the plate is round, you see that it is round by seeing that it projects an elliptical perspectival-shape (P-shape) and by understanding that the P-shape would change in characteristic ways if you were to move in relation to the plate. But colors, unlike shapes, it would seem, are themselves looks. This would seem to make apparent colors the looks of looks, a notion that is probably not coherent. The problem, at base, is this: If colors, in contrast with shapes, are ways things look, then it is not possible to explain our experience of the actual color of a thing in terms of looks, in the way that we were able to explain the experience of the actual shape of a thing in terms of our experience of how it looks (its P-shape) from here. For the way a thing looks with respect to color from here is just another experience of color. There is nothing, it would seem, that stands to color as P-properties (perspectival shape and perspectival size) stand to their corresponding properties.

The qualia theory would seem to be at an advantage here. It holds that for something to look red to someone is for it to give rise to an experience with a certain qualitative or sensational property. Its looking red consists in the fact that it gives rise to that qualitative state in a person. Apparent colors, on this view, are what Peacocke (1983) called sensational properties of experience, namely, properties of what it is like to have the experience that are not (really) properties the experience presents the world as having.

The qualia theory proposes that apparent colors are qualia that we encounter in having an experience. We have already noticed that this theory is tangled up with the possibilities of zombies and inverted spectra. The qualia theory raises other metaphysical puzzles as well. Jackson (1982, 1986), for example, has argued that qualia are not physical: You can know all the physical facts there are and still not know what it is like to see something red, what it is like to make the acquaintance of *that* quale.

However problematic these consequences of the qualia theory may or may not be, the qualia theory is widely thought, even by critics (such as Pettit), to have the virtue of phenomenological plausibility. The qualia theorist grants that how we represent the world as being in our experience shapes what it is like to have an experience. But, he or she insists, there are also aspects of what it is like to have an experience (e.g., of redness) that are not aspects of how the experience presents the world as being.

These further determiners of the character of consciousness are qualia. When we see that something is red, according to this theory, we do so on the basis of the experience to which the seen object gives rise in us.

But is the qualia theory phenomenologically apt? Does this picture cohere with a plausible account of what experience—in particular, color experience—is in fact like? There are reasons to doubt that it is.

One ground for skepticism concerns what I call the atomicity problem. Experiences are ineliminably holistic in a sense that can be made tolerably precise. What you are given in experience is always a structured field. You are never given individual, atom-like qualia.

Consider your impression of the detailed scene in front of you. As discussed in chapter 2, it does not seem to you as if all the detail is represented in your consciousness. You don't take yourself to see it all at once. The detail is visually present thanks to your possession of the skills that enable you to reach out and grasp the detail as you need it. What you experience, then, outstrips what you are strictly aware of now, or what you are attending to now. Crucially, you can no more grasp *the whole scene* in consciousness all at once than see all sides of the tomato at once, or the occluded parts of the cat behind the fence.

At least some perceptual content is, in this sense, *virtual* content. It is present in the way that the information on a remote server is present on your desktop. It is present thanks to your possession of the skills needed to acquire the relevant information at will.

But the computer network metaphor breaks down. In the computer network case, we can contrast what is genuinely represented on your desktop computer with what is represented only virtually with the help of dynamic links to a remote server. The content of experience, I would like to argue, is virtual *all the way in*. Notice that although the whole facing surface of the tomato is present to you, in contrast with the far side, which is out of view, you can no more embrace the *whole* of the facing side at once in consciousness than embrace the *whole* tomato in consciousness all at once. This is clear on reflection, I think. Further evidence comes from work on change blindness. In a recent demonstration conducted by Kevin O'Regan (mentioned in chapter 2), the color of the object you are staring at changes *while you examine it*. So long as attention is not directed to color in particular, perceivers tend not to notice even such a patent and gross change as this!

This shows that we cannot factor experience into an *occurrent* and a *merely virtual* or *potential* part. Experience is fractal, in this sense. At any level of analysis, it always presents a structured field that extends outward to a periphery, with elements that are out of view. There is always room, within experience, for shifts of attention.

The point is this: A perceptual experience doesn't analyze or break down into the experience of atomic elements, or simple features. Experience is always of a field, with structure, and you can never comprehend the whole field in a single act of consciousness. Something always remains present, but out of view. All you can do is run through features serially. But the moment you stop and try to make a specific feature the sole object of your consideration—*this shade of red*, for example—it slips away from you in the sense that it exceeds what you can take in, in completeness, at an instant. This is true even of a *Ganzfeld*. Suppose you are in a giant grey fog. Nothing visually distinguishes here from there. And yet, you are not given a simple property when you are in such a situation. The grey is spread out in space. There's the grey up there, and the grey down here. You can't grasp it all at once.

Qualities are available in experience as possibilities, as potentialities, but not as givens. Experience is a dynamic process of navigating the pathways of these possibilities. Experience depends on the skills needed to make one's way.

In the present context, the upshot of this is important. According to the qualia theory, qualia are meant to be the experienced determiners of the qualitative character of experience that are independent of the way the experience presents things to you as being. The distinctive redness of red is, on this view, fixed by (or perhaps identical to) the particular quale that is encountered when one sees something of the relevant shade of red. But this conception of qualia is vulnerable.

Consider: If what I have said about the structured field of experience is true, then there can be nothing in experience answering to the demands placed on qualia. For there is no experiential quality—however simple, however evident—that is such that we can encompass it completely within a moment of consciousness. Every quale will have *qualities*, only some of which can be contemplated at a given time.

One way to put the qualitative predicament is in terms of a regress. Because there are no simples in experience, every quality has further qualities. Positing qualia then leads to an infinite regress. For you can always inquire after the qualia you enjoy when contemplating any of your qualia!

Such an approach might seem easy to dismiss. When you look at a red tomato, or a blue shirt, you enjoy a quality and that quality is simply there in your consciousness and it is there quite apart from your knowledge or beliefs about color. This response is suggested by Galen Strawson (1989), who has claimed, that the idea of color qualia—of the qualitative character of color experience—can be taken for granted.[4] He writes: "Most . . . will agree that the notion of the qualitative character of colour-experience can reasonably be taken for granted. And for present purposes, a sufficient reply to those who disagree is simple, as follows. Consider your present visual experience. Look at the bookshelf. (Get out some of the brightest books.) There you have it" (Strawson 1989, 194).

The trouble with this line of thought, so it seems to me, is that when I look at a book and attend to its color, I don't see something simple, I see something complex. The red is partly cast in shadow, say, and it has bits of orange in it, and here the texture of the book's cloth seems to permeate the color of the cover. The book's color stands out strikingly against the blue background of my desk. Where, in this temporally extended episode of attentive exploration of the book, do I encounter the quale of redness?

The point of all this is not that it *proves* that the qualia theory is wrong. I haven't done this. After all, the qualia theorist can posit qualia for holistic states, or processes whereby experiential molecules are generated by the combination of qualitative atoms. My aim is less ambitious: to call into question whether the qualia theory is really so phenomenologically apt.

One reason the experience of color generates the atomicity problem has to do with the well-understood fact that colors form a system. Any two determinate colors stand in determinate relations with respect to lightness, hue, and saturation. The red of my copy of the *Tractatus*, for example, may be darker than and more saturated than the blue of my shirt. Any two determinate colors will stand in relations of similarity along these dimensions. Colors stand in other sorts of relations as well. The blue of my shirt may be distinctly reddish, while the red of my copy of the *Tractatus* may have no perceptible amount of any other color in it. This difference between so-called unique and binary colors is an important feature of the way colors are phenomenally organized. In addition, there are other kinds of similarities and differences. Red is more like yellow, as a rule, than it is like blue, and blue is more like green than it is like red.

The status of these relations among colors is complex and controversial. For example, one might be inclined to believe that these phenomenal relations among colors are *necessary*. There is no possible world, so it might seem, in which orange is not reddish-yellow, and there's no possible world in which yellow isn't more like orange than it is like green. Alternatively, one might think (as Wittgenstein apparently did at one stage) that facts such as these are *formal*; they pertain to color given the "logical grammar" of color vocabulary, and they hold independent of the fact that real colored objects have the sorts of complex aspect profiles described in section 4.2. If the fact that a surface darkens as it falls in shadow is a fact about *object* color, the fact that red and yellow are elements of orange is a constitutive fact about what orange *is* (about color per se).

Whatever one says about these themes—for a review, see Thompson 1995 and Hardin 1986—their significance for the present discussion is as follows: The significant point is not merely that color qualia stand in relations of similarity. Nor is the point that color qualities—such as the red of my book—are in part constituted by their location in formal color space. Rather, the point is that our experience of colors is shaped by our implicit grasp on their positions in color space. We experience them as imbued with possibilities of variation, as possessing degrees of freedom in a space of phenomenal possibilities. We don't *see* the rest of color space when seeing the red look of the book. But our sense of the presence of that larger color space contributes to what is like when we experience red.

The upshot of these considerations is that to experience even this particular reddish look of the car in this light, one must grasp and draw on one's grasp of its relations to other colors. This puts pressure on the idea that color experience can be analyzed into the experience of atoms of color consciousness such as qualia are supposed to be.

4.4   Enacting How Things Look

In what, then, does the experience of the red look of the book consist, if not in one's acquaintance with a simple quality of experience, namely, the red quale?

To approach this question, let us ask another and see if we can answer it. Is it really true, as the qualia theory would have it, that color experience is independent of our possession of discriminatory capacities, that is, capacities to pick out, sift, and track objects on the basis of their color? There must surely be something wrong with a behaviorism that insists that something's looking red to one consists just in one's ability to discriminate it. After all, when we visually discriminate red things, picking them out, say, from among green ones, we do so on the basis of how they look! Discriminatory behavior flows from discriminating experience; one needs a nonbehaviorist account of what it is for something to look red.

Nevertheless, I think we can question whether we really understand what it would be to experience a color quality in the absence of such skills. Consider that colors, as discussed in section 4.3, stand in a range of apparently necessary relations to one another. To perceive something as looking red, here and now, say, is to perceive it as standing in a complex set of relationships of similarity and difference. To perceive such a quality, therefore, is already to be in possession of and to be able to exercise a range of discriminatory capacities.

This isn't meant to be a logical point. It is underwritten by our phenomenology. It is by no means obvious that one could *experience* something as, say, looking a particular shade of orange, without being able, thereby, to discriminate it as different from something green, or, more subtly, as more yellow than something only red, and as lighter than a dark shade of blue. One way to get at this is that *the way* we discriminate colors is precisely in terms of their phenomenal similarities and differences with other colors. For this reason, I think, only one who possesses such a battery of discriminatory skills could experience something as looking colored in this way or another.

This sort of consideration may lie behind Pettit's proposal that what it is to experience something as looking red is to experience it as looking such as to enable you to make certain discriminations. He writes, "The object looks red so far as it overtly enables you to sift and sort and track it in the red-appropriate manner, and to make corresponding judgments; it looks red so far as you see it as extracting those responses from you" (2003a, 230). Or to use a manner of speaking he also deploys: it is to see the object as looking such as to enable you to make various discriminations.

At first blush, it might seem that this proposal will be open to the charge of behaviorism. After all, it seems to analyze *looking red* in terms of discriminatory behaviors. But it is far from obvious that this charge can be made to stick, for the charge may rest on an overly simplistic account of the discriminatory capacities in question. The brute ability to sift red and green things, for example, is much too coarse-grained to count as a necessary condition of one's experiencing something as looking red, say. However, the ability to experience something as lighter than this, as darker than that, as more like this in respect of hue than like that, although more like that in respect of brightness than like this, tracks very well the quality of the redness in question. To experience something as a determinate shade of green, say, is to experience it as disposed to blend in, in one background, and to jump out against a different background. Indeed, it is to experience it as blending in *this way*, among these lighter greens, but as blending in, say, *in a very different way*—becoming invisible, fading from view, getting lost, etc.—among these other green things.

Of such a mature range of discriminatory capacities it does indeed seem reasonable to say that to experience something as looking such as to enable one to make a range of discriminations—to see it as provoking different possible saliencies in these ways—is to experience it as looking a particular shade of red. The key is that the discriminatory capacities in question, if they are to be more than mere external evidence of color experience, need to possess not only the multiplicity of the essential relations of phenomenal color space, but also the multiplicity of color aspect profiles.

Having thus elaborated Pettit's account, let us attempt to answer his question, the one that began this section. How does a thing that looks red look? If we are using "looks red" to refer to the way it looks here and now and not as a judgment about its overall aspect profile (i.e., about its actual color), then we can say the following: To look red is to look such as to allow one to pick it out from green things in these various ways (in the "red appropriate" ways), from pink things in those ways, and so forth.

However, we can go further than this. When something looks a determinate red, here and now, it looks, here and now, as if it has a distinctive color aspect profile. In just this same way, for a round plate to look elliptical from here is for it to look, from here, as if it were elliptical. Now we can individuate its elliptical appearance, as I have suggested, in terms of

P-properties. But we can also say that it is for the plate to look, from here, as if it *is* elliptical, to look as if its profile would change not in the round-thing way, but in the elliptical-thing way. We are smart enough to balance these two different interpretations of how things look at once. Take a fire engine. It looks red; that is, it looks such that it would vary in appearance in a range of comprehensible ways, given the color aspect profile of the relevant red. It also looks red here and now, that is, looks such as to afford opportunities for contrast *like so* with other objects and qualities. In looking so, however, it also looks the way, from here, a red thing would look, namely, like a thing whose appearance would vary in appropriate ways.

It is possible, then, to bring the account of color into accord with the earlier account of shape. A round thing looks elliptical from here when it cuts such and such a figure on a suitably selected occlusion plane. This sort of cutting of a figure can be understood in sensorimotor terms. It is for a thing to look *like this* (said while pointing with one's hand and moving it appropriately). A similar story can be told about some red thing's looking dark red from here, that is, its agreement in color with *this* sample in these conditions. Take the example of the sun-dappled wall again. You see it is uniformly white, but you also see that here it matches a grey chip like this (say, here and now), and there the wall matches a different chip. In this way we give content to the idea of its looking one way rather than another with respect to color from here in these conditions. Crucially, as we have already seen, the account of how it looks is to be spelled out in terms of a repertoire of discriminatory capacities.

Are these discriminatory capacities sensorimotor capacities? In our extended sense of sensorimotor capacity, yes. That is, they are, if you like, ways of understanding color change, movement in a qualitative space of color. They may also be sensorimotor capacities in our first movement-dependent sense, namely, knowledge of the way sensory stimulation changes as we move. For how things look from here, now, is in part a function of the way things stimulate me now, and the way this stimulation varies as eyes move. These subtle changes are subpersonal, to be sure, and so they are, as far as consciousness is concerned, inscrutable. But they are changes in us brought about by our contact with the world, and they are changes that, plausibly, we implicitly understand. Indeed, as O'Regan and Noë (2001a) have argued, this very fact partly explains why color qualia (such as they are) are seemingly ineffable and mysterious. We only have conscious access to certain aspects of their sensorimotor profile.

4.5 Phenomenal Objectivism

The enactive theory of color experience suggests an account of the nature of color. The color of an object is a way its appearance varies as relevant conditions change, for example, as ambient light darkens over the course of a day, or as the source of illumination moves, or as the object moves from one sort of lighting (say, daylight) into a different sort (e.g., moonlight, or firelight). Colors are ways colored things change their appearance as color-critical conditions change.

Colors are patterns of organization in how things look. They *are* looks. This way of putting things gives a nod to the traditional distinction between primary and secondary qualities. The apparent shape of an object is determined by its actual shape insofar as how it looks with respect to shape from here depends on its actual shape. Very few thinkers have been tempted by the phenomenalist suggestion that the actual shape *is* the way the thing changes apparent shape as vantage point varies. The actual shape, after all, is a way of filling out space, whereas the apparent shape is an appearance or look; it is how such a thing looks from here. The phenomenalist account is wrongheaded when it comes to shape, but it is exactly right, I propose, as an account of color. The color of an object is just the way its apparent color changes as viewing conditions change.

The shape of a thing is independent of its look or feel in a way that the color of a thing isn't independent of its look. For this reason, it is possible to give an account of shape that is independent of an account of apparent shape, but it is impossible to give an account of color that is independent of an account of *apparent* color. This difference between shape and color is the basis of an influential philosophical tradition regarding the nature of color: Colors, according to this tradition, are dispositions (powers or tendencies) of objects to look (e.g., red, blue, etc.) to a perceiver. For example, Newton wrote: "[T]he Rays to speak properly are not coloured. In them there is nothing else than a certain Power and Disposition to stir up a Sensation of this or that Colour . . . So Colours in the object are nothing but a Disposition to reflect this or that sort of Rays more copiously than the rest" ([1704] 1952).

According to this view, to be red, for example, is to be such as to look red to normal perceivers in normal lighting conditions. The qualia theory of color can be thought of as providing dispositionalism with the means to avoid the threatening circularity: To experience something as red is to experience it as producing a certain characteristic quale in one, a quale whose intrinsic nature is knowable independent of settling the question of object color. Red things are those that give rise to experiences with a certain sensational property we have come to associate with redness (Peacocke 1983).

Is it true that red things are those that are disposed to look red to normal perceivers in normal circumstances, as the dispositionalist contends? On an innocuous interpretation of this statement, it is indeed, and what makes it true is the fact that a suitably placed normal perceiver can usually tell, by looking, that a presented red object is red. It looks red in the sense that one can tell by looking that it is red. This innocuous interpretation, however, is compatible with its being the case that *how the red thing looks* varies greatly as viewing conditions change and so with its being the case that there isn't any *one* determinate apparent color that is the apparent color of a given red thing (Putnam 1999, 39–40). If there are qualia, then, it would follow, there isn't any one quale that is the looks-effect, as it were, of things even of a determinate shade of red. The point is not merely that the red thing won't look red, say, in green light. Presumably artificial green lighting won't count as a "normal condition" of viewing. I have in mind such facts as, to be very specific, that when you get up to reach for the knife to slice the tomato, and your body casts it in shadow, the tomato visibly darkens in color; that when your companion turns on a second light in the kitchen the tomato visibly brightens, perhaps revealing surface irregularities that consist in part in differences in color; and so on. Importantly, these are changes in the way a thing looks *in normal conditions*. The innocuous interpretation is thus compatible with a second interpretation according to which it is false that red things (i.e., things of a determinate color) are disposed to look one and the same way, with respect to color, in a range of conditions that we can reasonably think of as normal. There is no single way that a thing looks when it looks even a determinate shade of red. However we understand the statement that red things are disposed to look red, it is important to stress that this statement lends no support to the qualia theory as an account of color experience.

The enactive account agrees with traditional dispositionalism that colors are dispositions or powers, but it disagrees with the traditional view about what sort of dispositions colors are. Colors, on the traditional view, are, crudely put, ways in which things give rise to experiences with a certain kind of quale in perceivers. Colors, on the enactive view, in contrast, are ways things are disposed to change their appearance as color-critical conditions change. That an object has a given color (say, a specific shade of red) is a fact about the way that object affects its environment (as has been argued by Broackes [1992], whose view anticipates much in the account that I present here). An object with a determinate color *acts on*, or *responds to*, its environment in a special way. For instance, it grows darker in a characteristic way in shadow, and it becomes brownish in green light; it stands out among blue things, in the characteristic way in which red things will stand out among blue things, but get lost among these red things, and so forth. It responds to illumination and background color in a very different way from this other pink object, and in subtly different ways from this other red one. To be a particular red is to bring about these sorts of apparent changes in how things look. To perceive something as red is to perceive it as thus acting on and capable of acting on its visible environment. In this way, the enactive view is an account of what it is to be red in terms of the *phenomenally salient ways* in which the object *interacts with* its environment.

This account of what it is to *be* a particular red is thus coordinated with our account of what it is to *experience something as* this shade of red. You experience it as this shade of red when you *understand* the way its appearance changes as color-critical conditions change, and you are able to experience its (merely) apparent color in *these conditions*, say, when you are able to see the thing as looking such as to enable you to differentiate it in ways that correspond to its aspect profile. In this way, the account of color I offer here treats colors as irreducibly phenomenal, but it avoids the circularity of saying that red things are those that *look red*.

This account of color explains a crucial fact about color and also an apparent paradox. The crucial fact is that colors are not merely visible; they are, in essence, *visibilia*. You do not, cannot, know what red is, say, if you haven't seen something red (although it is possible to find out that something is red without seeing it). The apparent paradox is this: Despite the fact that colors are visibilia, there is a distinction that can be drawn, in the domain of color, between appearance and reality. A red object can look (merely appear to be) brown in certain lighting. Its looking brown here and now doesn't make it brown. The phenomenal account of color I am suggesting can explain this appearance/reality contrast. Red things, on this view, are precisely the sort of things that look brown under these lighting conditions. That they do is given in their color aspect profile.

4.6 Color Belongs to the Environment

The color of a surface is its disposition to change its appearance as relevant viewing conditions change. Color, therefore, is intrinsically phenomenal. This fact, however, does not make color "unreal," or merely "subjective." Colors are dispositions of objects to act on and interact with the environment in determinate ways. Color is relational, but it is not the sort of relational property traditional dispositionalism, such as that of Newton, had in mind. According to that dispositionalism, as we have noted, colors are tendencies to give rise to qualitative states in perceivers. On the view I am developing, in contrast, colors are ways objects act on and are affected by the environment. Colors, on this view, have a status that is similar to apparent shapes and sizes: The color a thing appears to have, like its apparent shape and size, varies as our relation to the thing varies, and as its relation to its environment changes. Colors, like all appearances, are genuine features of the environment.

To say that colors belong to the environment is to say, among other things, that they are, in ways that I will try to make clear, objective. Their objectivity has been challenged in different ways by different theorists. Some philosophers claim that colors (and other appearances) lack objectivity because they can only be perceived from a particular point of view—that is to say, the sort of point of view available to those with our particular kind of visual system. There are two reasons to doubt this claim. First, it may not be true that colors are only perceivable from one point of view. It *is* true that colors are visible qualities; you can't touch or smell them (synesthesia and its puzzles aside). But there are good reasons to believe that you don't have to have a perceptual system like those of adult humans to perceive colors. Bees perceive color, as do fish, and birds, but there are many respects in which their visual systems are different from ours. Certainly, there is no obvious sense in which, in virtue of having vision, bees, humans, birds, and fish have *the same* point of view.

Work on "sensory substitution" (as discussed in chapters 1 and 3) suggests that it may be possible to *see* (as we do) without even having a visual system. At the current time, no sensory substitution system supports color vision. But there is nothing in the nature of color that rules out this artificial color vision in principle. We can wonder what substance can be given to the claim that the prosthetic perceiver (using a sensory substitution system such as TVSS) and the normal visual perceiver really occupy the *same* point of view.[5]

There is a second reason to doubt that the fact that the only way to know colors is to see them entails that colors are lacking in objectivity. From its being the case that it is only possible to encounter (perceive, experience, come to know) colors in a given modality, it does not follow that colors are themselves *existence-dependent* on the possession of that modality by perceivers. A world in which nothing occupied the visual point of view would be a world in which there were no experiences of color; but it would not, thereby, be a world in which there were no colors.

Different species differ in their perceptual capacities. Dogs can detect odors that are undetectable by humans. Humans can see colors that are undetectable by animals such as dogs. Pigeons, in turn, are pentachromats (having five different wavelength-sensitive cones) and may perceive colors that humans cannot perceive. This raises fascinating empirical/methodological questions such as, for example, How can we investigate what pigeons can experience?, and important philosophical questions such as, What would it be to be a color and yet not one of the colors that we can see? (A detailed discussion of these can be found in Thompson 1995.) The crucial point here is that the fact that there are qualities perceivable by pigeons that we cannot perceive, or that there are qualities we can perceive that dogs cannot, is not in itself a reason for doubting the independent reality of these qualities. If all sentient beings were to disappear off the face of the earth tomorrow, then there would be no color experiences tomorrow. But there would be colors.

Hardin (1986) and others have challenged this, arguing that at least a range of color phenomena *reduce to* neurophysiological phenomena. The fact that there is no such thing as reddish green, and that green afterimages occur after looking at red patches—examples of what is known as color opponency—are explained by facts about the way the visual system responds to light at differing wavelengths. In particular, it is believed that postreceptoral processing of color is organized into three "opponent" channels, the red-green, blue-yellow, and black-white (or chromatic/achromatic) channels. Color opponency is explained by the fact that activation of the red process requires, as a matter of neural architecture, the corresponding *de*activation of the green process. Nothing can be reddish-green, because nothing can simultaneously activate the red and green processes (see Hurvich 1981 for the details; also Hardin 1986; Thompson 1995).

I am inclined to doubt that these considerations force us to deny the objective existence of colors. It isn't really clear whether the fact that there is no such thing as reddish-green is *explained* by the facts of human visual processing of color. One might think that there is no reddish-green for the same reason that there is no light black. That there is no reddish-green is a necessary truth about the nature of redness and greenness. The point is not merely that nothing *is* reddish-green—what would be a fact about our environment—but that, given the *systematic* nature of color (discussed in section 4.3) reddish-green is impossible, in very much the way that, say, real numbers are impossible within the system of the integers. Structurally speaking, red is too distant from green to be *co-present* with it. When we say of orange that it is a mixture of red and yellow, what we mean, intuitively, is that there is a process of adding yellow successively to red, such that you first get yellowish-red, then reddish-yellow, and finally, pure yellow. (Crucially, we are speaking here of *phenomenal* color, not of pigments or lights.) But there is no analogous sense in which you pass through binary red-green on your way to some other color. Red can yellow, and it can become successively bluer, but it must become yellow or blue *before* it can become green.

Hardin cites Crane and Piantinida (1983), who report an experimental condition in which subjects reported seeing reddish-green and bluish-yellow. The experiment turned on stabilizing the projection of a boundary between a red and a green patch on the retina. Krauskopf (1963) showed that a stabilized boundary would provoke filling in: If the boundary between a red disk and a green annulus were stabilized, the entire large disk (formed by merging the two) would come to be perceived as green. This is frequently explained on the supposition that information from the exterior boundary is used to "fill in" the extended interior of the disk. In Crane and Piantinida's setup, some subjects reported seeing the region surrounding a stabilized boundary as the binary color "reddish-green." Billock, Gleason, and Tsou (2001) have recently replicated Crane and Piantinida's finding. Sophisticated subjects (psychophysicists, psychologists) all report experiences of genuine, "forbidden" colors. If these findings are to be taken at face value, they certainly call into question the claim that there is no such color as reddish-green. And they lend support to the idea that properties of colors depend on features of our nervous system.

There are strong reasons for caution in regard to Crane and Piantinida's and Billock, Gleason and Tsou's findings. As we noticed in sections 2.8 and 3.3, the fact that perceivers may be strongly inclined to characterize themselves as seeing a contour, for example, when presented with an illusory contour, does not show that they are in a state qualitatively indistinguishable from that of genuinely seeing a contour. (Compare figures 2.7 and 2.8.). With this in mind, we can grant that the experiments in question set up unusual circumstances in which subjects are strongly and genuinely disposed *to say that they see reddish-green*. The question is whether they are strongly disposed *to* say this because, in fact, they have an experience as of reddish-green, or simply because they have an experience they find it natural to describe in this way. This is not an idle speculation. Perceptual effects created by stablizing images on the retina are effects that, by the very nature of the case, are delicate, tenuous, and difficult to maintain. It would be hasty just to dismiss the studies out of hand. In light of considerations such as these, however, it is very difficult to know how much weight to give them.

Whatever we say about cases such as these, I am skeptical of Hardin's neuropsychological reductionism about color. We can grant that our ability to experience colors depends, in the way Hardin describes, on our possession of the requisite perceptual (and neural) systems. All that follows from this is that our possession of these prerequisites is necessary for us to enjoy the sort of experience we do. Facts about our sensory systems determine the kinds of experiences we can have. Further argument would be needed to show that colors are therefore dependent on us for their existence or nature.

Traditional dispositionalists deny the objectivity of color by arguing that colors are psychological. This is a further sense in which color is thought to be subjective. Palmer, for example, writes:

People universally believe that objects *look* colored because they *are* colored, just as we experience them: The sky looks blue because it *is* blue, grass looks green because it *is* green, and blood looks red because it *is* red . . . As surprising as it may seem, these beliefs are fundamentally mistaken. Neither objects nor lights are actually "colored" in anything like the way we experience them. Rather, color is a *psychological* property of our visual experiences when we look at objects and lights, not a *physical* property of those objects and lights. (1999a, 95)

Colors, in other words, are sensations or, in Peacocke's terminology, sensational properties of experiences. Colors are not properties of objects, because they are, in effect, *in us*. Color is an effect of light on our nervous system (Palmer 1999a; Hardin 1986; Hurvich 1981). Colors are unreal; color *experiences* are real.

If even a small bit of the forgoing argument is right, it should be clear that nothing forces us to accept this conclusion. On the account of colors offered here, colors are not sensations. Phenomenal objectivism recognizes that colors, like other sensory appearances, depend on causal relations. But colors are not relations between objects and the nervous system. Rather, they depend on relations between objects and viewing conditions. There is nothing *sensation-dependent* or *experiential* about these relations themselves. Nor is there anything about relational (versus nonrelational or intrinsic) properties that makes them unreal or ontologically secondary. (Shaquille O'Neill has the relational property of being taller than Lance Armstrong. Although a relation between Shaquille and Lance, Shaquille's being taller than Lance is a genuine property of Shaquille.)

Colors are objective in yet a further sense: Frege wrote that "what is objective . . . is what is subject to laws, what can be conceived and judged, what is expressible in words. What is purely intuitable is not communicable" ([1884] 1950, 35). Colors are objective by this criterion as well. Statements of color—such as "the red of that car is brighter than the red of that ball," "this is red," "if you mix a green pigment with a red pigment, you will get a colorless, grey/black pigment"—express thoughts that may be communicated and evaluated for truth or falsity. These are *facts* about color.

It is widely believed that qualia (say, in contrast with colors) are *not* objective in this sense. They are, as Frege himself believed, merely intuitable, private sensations. It is not possible to "communicate" my sensation of red to you, any more than it is possible for you to have my headache. If you have it, then it is not mine. Supporters of the qualia theory hold that although you and I might agree that this car is red, that it has the same color as that building, and so forth, it might nevertheless be the case that the color quale I enjoy in looking at it is unlike that which you enjoy in looking at it. This difference in the character of our experiences is not something we can communicate. (This is the inverted spectrum hypothesis, once again.)

A full discussion of this question is beyond what I can accomplish here. For reasons given earlier, I am inclined to think that it is an illusion that there are qualia in this sense. The ineffability of color appearances may stem, in large measure, from the fact that how a thing looks, here and now, with respect to color, is *very complex*. Its looking a determinate shade of red, for example, is a matter of its looking such as to enable one to discriminate it in a *very* broad range of different ways, it is to experience it as possessing a complicated network of potential saliencies. This ineffability does not make it impossible to make statements that are determinate in regard to truth about color and color appearance. It only rules out the possibility of, as it were, transmitting color experiences by verbal devices.

I have emphasized that there are several senses in which color may be thought of as objective: Colors are not sensations; they are relational, but they are not relations between things and the mind, but between things and their environments; colors are not existent-dependent on perceivers (or their sensory systems); colors may be the intentional objects of thought and of intersubjective communication. I close this section with two senses in which perhaps we ought to concede that color is not objective.

First, there is considerable disagreement among "normal" perceivers about colors. If you are given the task of picking out pure green (i.e., green with no traces of blue or yellow in it), from among a pile of color chips, there is a good chance that you will be able to decide, with confidence, which chip is pure green. But it turns out that normal perceivers disagree rather widely on which chip is pure green. My pure green may look distinctly bluish to you. (This is discussed in Hardin 1986.)

It's worth noting that the fact that blue looks one way to me and another way to you does not entail that there isn't a fact of the matter about how it looks simpliciter. "Ruby Tuesday" may sound like a Rolling Stones song to me, and a Beatles song to you, but that doesn't mean that, as a matter of fact, it sounds like neither.

Second, colors are perceiver-dependent in a sense we haven't yet considered. Dennett (1991) and Thompson (1995) have argued that, in a historical/evolutionary sense, the existence of colorful things is an evolutionary response to the coevolution of color-sensitive beings. There would not be color in the natural world if there were no color-sensitive perceivers. Color functions ecologically as a signal for such features as (as noticed by Gibson 1979, 98) ripeness (fruit), poisonousness (plants and arachnids), fertility (flowers, orangutans). In addition, colors play an important role in object discrimination and concealment. These traits would never have evolved in the biological world if not for the *co*evolution of color sensitivity. This provides a striking, albeit rather singular, sense in which color is *perceiver-dependent* and so, in that sense, subjective rather than autonomous. In any event, it seems clear that this story can't hold for all instances of color in nature, however. Rubies would be red, and the sky blue, regardless of whether there were sentient color perceivers.

4.7   Is Color Physical?

Colors, on the enactive account, are real. Colors are visible properties of, for example, surfaces. In particular, colors are ways objects interact with their environments, especially illumination. They are patterns in how things look.

I have been defending the view from attack by dispositionalists and others who deny that color is real because they hold that color is subjective (e.g., a kind of sensation). Color, according to these theories, is *in us*, not *in the world*.

But phenomenal objectivism is also vulnerable to criticism by color *realists* who believe that colors are physical (as opposed to phenomenal or environmental) properties of surfaces. The best developed version of color physicalism holds that color is *surface spectral reflectance*, namely, that property by virtue of which an object is disposed to reflect a given proportion of incident light at each wavelength in the visible spectrum (Byrne and Hilbert 2003). Physicalism offers an account of colors as objective in all the ways the enactive account treats them as objective: They are sensation-independent, and they are independent of the existence of perceivers. The physicalist picture, *like that of the phenomenal objectivist,* but unlike that of the subjectivist, accommodates nicely such facts as that we experience the redness of the tomato as a property *of the tomato* and that, when we look at three tomatoes that are the same color, we take it that the tomatoes share a property in common. Physicalism would also seem to be able to account elegantly for the basic facts of color constancy. The spectral composition of the light reflected off the tomato differs greatly in the garden, under the fluorescent lighting in the kitchen, and in the refrigerator. What does not change in these different conditions of illumination is the proportion of incident light at each wavelength of the visible spectrum that the object is disposed to reflect. It is this constant state—the object's surface spectral reflectance—that grounds the relative constancy of color despite changing conditions of illumination.

The physicalist, moreover, can accept the enactive claim that colors are ways objects act on illumination. But the physicalist insists that it is possible to characterize the *ways* objects affect incident light in purely physical (that is to say, nonphenomenal) terms. Is this true?

The trouble with the proposal that colors are surface spectral reflectances (SSRs) is that it grounds the *objectivity* of color at the cost of the *phenomenality* of color (a point made by several writers, e.g., Hardin 1986; Johnston 1992; Thompson 1995). For the physicalist, being red isn't a matter of looking a certain way, it's a matter of having a disposition differentially to reflect light at different wavelengths. There is nothing intrinsically phenomenal about color, on this view. Indeed, on this view it will not even generally be the case that colors are visible.

This is revealed by considering the existence of *metameric pairs*, that is, objects that look to be (and so, pretheoretically speaking, are) the same color relative to a range of conditions of illumination, but that differ in surface spectral reflectance (and that thus differ in the way they would act on physical light). For any given object, of any given SSR, there will be an indefinite number of other objects with different SSRs that nevertheless tend to look the same in a broad range of conditions. Metamerism is a consequence of the fact that all information about the spectral composition of light reaching the eyes is mediated by the activity of three different kinds of cones. Cones are affected by light of different wavelengths in an identical manner, although cones differ in their probability of firing in response to photons of one wavelength or another. The activity of a long wavelength cone alone, therefore, does not carry information about whether the light stimulating it is of long wavelength, or, say, high-intensity medium wavelength. As a result, one and the same activity pattern of receptors can be produced by light of an indefinite number of different spectral compositions. This in turn guarantees that objects with radically different reflectance profiles can have the same effect on the nervous system.

Given metamerism, physicalists must reckon that objects that look the same with respect to color could actually be different in color (because they differ in SSR). Indeed, they must acknowledge that for every determinate shade we can perceive, there are an indefinitely large number of *different colors* that are *perceptually indistinguishable* from the given one. These color differences are invisible. Color vision, it would seem, is at best a very poor guide to object color.

Byrne and Hilbert (1997, 2003) propose to deal with this apparent shortcoming of the physicalist view as follows: Determinate colors, they argue, just like color *categories* (such as red and blue), are not identical to numerically distinct SSRs, but rather, to *types* of SSRs. Two objects can thus be the very same shade of red even though they disagree in their SSR, because each SSR is an SSR of the same type. Which type? Presumably the type that tends, under a range of circumstances, to look the same way to normal perceivers. The members of the SSR type that constitute a given shade of red may not have much else in common; as Byrne and Hilbert say, it may be an uninteresting class from a physical point of view. This shows that colors are *anthropocentric* in the sense that their existence is of interest only because we have the sorts of perceptual systems that we do in fact have. That colors are anthropocentric, however, doesn't detract from the fact that they are real and, moreover, that they are physical. Information about how things look plays a role in *picking out SSR types*, but the colors (SSR types) that are thus picked out are objects whose nature (and existence) is independent of how things look to us. Thus modified, the color physicalist is able to defend the claim that metameric pairs are indeed of the same color, even though their SSRs differ. Color physicalism is preserved by making colors sets of SSRs.

This modification is enough to ensure that color vision is a good guide to how things are with respect to color. But does it preserve the intuition that color is phenomenal? One might doubt this. The thought that colors are phenomenal goes beyond the mere claim that they are visible; the thought is that colors are intrinsically visual (phenomenal). One way to bring this out is by observing that you wouldn't *have the concept red* (you wouldn't know what red is) if you took it to be the concept whose application was warranted when and only when a thing had a certain SSR. For what such a *conception* would leave out is the fact that one who understands *red* is one who can apply it to an object because of a feature of the way it looks. Any view that identifies colors with physical properties of surfaces has to give up the claim that colors are phenomenal in this sense.

Hardin (1986), Broackes (1992), Thompson (1995), and others have questioned whether there can be a physicalist account of the phenomenal relations that hold among the colors (e.g., the uniqueness/binary distinction, similarity relations in general, the facts of color opponency). After all, the dimensions along which color vary are three, but the dimensions along which ratios of incident to reflected light at different wavelengths can vary is infinite.

As Thompson puts it: "There is no mapping from the reflectance colour space to phenomenal colour space that is structure-preserving in a robust sense and that does not proceed through one of the perceiver-dependent, psychological or psychophysical colour spaces" (1995, 124).

Byrne and Hilbert (1997, 2003) have responded to these arguments, as has Tye (2000). I do not want to discuss the details of these responses here. Attempts to refine the physicalist position are, in the end, unmotivated. This becomes clear when we recognize, first, that the price of giving up the identification of colors and SSRs is *not* subjectivism about colors. For a phenomenal objectivist, what things of a given color have in common is the way they look. The redness isn't merely a physical property of the surface, nor is it a relation between the surface and the perceiver. It is a phenomenally salient relation between the surface and the environment. Second, not only can the phenomenal objectivism developed here account for color objectivity, but it can do so in a way that is *consistent* with the physical facts about object surface color that the physicalist adduces. In particular, phenomenal objectivists can agree, with the physicalist, that color is determined by SSR (in a wide range of cases, at least), in the sense that SSR is a preeminent causal factor determining how things look. But phenomenal objectivism can do something physicalism cannot do: It can give a natural account of why it is that things of radically different physical composition can, say, all be red. The redness is a fact about the way they vary in appearance as conditions change.

It's worth mentioning that the physicalist is forced to deny not only that colors are intrinsically phenomenal, but also that they are relational. Colors, according to the physicalism we are considering, are intrinsic properties of physical surfaces. A thing has whatever color it has independent of its relations to its surrounding environment. There is reason to doubt that this can be true, however (at least if we hold fast to the view that colors are phenomenal). How a thing looks with respect to color depends not only on its character (e.g., its propensity to reflect light and so to affect photoreceptors), but also on the character of surrounding objects. This is demonstrated by *simultaneous color contrast* (discussed in section 4.2). For example, a line might look dark grey against a light background and pinkish against a dark background, and the black of the leather jacket on television is, in fact, not different physically from the gray/green darkness of the television screen when it is off.

At the beginning of this section I mentioned that the SSR view was on strong ground when it comes to explaining color constancy. We don't experience variation in the color of a tomato as we take it indoors, despite the fact that the spectral composition of the light it reflects to the eyes changes radically, because, according to the physicalist, SSR does not change. What we track when we track color is SSR. The problem with this claim is that there *are* changes in color as conditions of illumination change. My point is not the familiar one, often repeated by psychologists, that color constancy breaks down or is only partial. The point rather is that perceptual content has dual aspects, as noted throughout chapters 3 and 4. The plate looks elliptical, and round, and the tomato looks the same *and different* with respect to color. Color changes under variations in illumination are perfectly noticeable, if we choose to attend to them. These changes are determinate. For example, you would indicate different color samples as the match to the brightly lit part of the wall and the part of the wall cast in shadow. We perceive the color as different, but we *discount* these differences, because we know that what interests us, in a broad range of cases, is not how the thing looks here and now, but how its look varies as conditions change (i.e., its color aspect profile). What we want is a view that allows us to comprehend how something that looks different can, in a sense, look the same. To account for this, we need a view that takes seriously that a thing's color depends constitutively on how it looks. If color is SSR, then how can we account for visible changes in color as conditions of illumination change?

4.8   Colors, Ecology, and the Phenomenal World

Can we really make sense of the idea that colors are objective but non-physical ways that objects affect their environment? One proposal, developed by Thompson (1995; Thompson, Palacios, and Varela 1992; see also Broackes 1992 and Noë 1995), is that the appropriate level at which to analyze color would be to view it as *ecological* in Gibson's sense. An ecological approach to color (as well as other appearances) treats it as *natural*, but as nonphysical.

As I discussed in chapter 3 (section 3.9), Gibson's ambient optic array can be thought of as the structured space of appearances. The sense of the Gibsonian claim that the ambient optic array specifies the environment is that how things look from here in these conditions specifies how they are, or rather, it does so for a suitably knowledgeable animal, one in possession of and ready to apply sensorimotor skill. But colors, at least on the view I have been defending, are themselves looks. An ecological account of color, therefore, will treat colors as ways objects act on the ambient optic array, namely, the light-filled, structured environment. Colors are not ways that objects affect light as the physicist might study it, or even light *as phenomenal* (as Broackes [1992], Westphal [1987], and Putnam [1992] have argued). It is the way they affect the light-filled environment.

If this account is right, then it introduces a kind of relativity into the account of color that is different from that which we have considered so far. Colors and other types of appearance, on an ecological approach, are genuine features of the environment. The environment, however, as Thompson (1995) explains, is not a neutral physical domain (see also Gibson 1979). Environments are codetermined by inhabitants of the environment. The environment is the physical world *as it is inhabited by the animal*. The perceptual world (the environment) is not a separate place or world; it is the world thought of from our standpoint (or from any animal's standpoint). It is our world.

This is an important idea, one we need to understand properly, especially in light of the forgoing discussion about objectivity. The perceptual world is not a subjective world. The perceptual world is not a world of effects produced in us—in our minds—by the actual world. But the perceptual world is the world *for us*. We can say that the world for us is not the physical world, in that it is not the world of items introduced and catalogued in physical theory. But it is the natural world (and perhaps also the cultural world). The ambient optic array is available to a creature who is equipped with a battery of sensory, motor, and cognitive capacities. It isn't that the perceptual world is *existence*-dependent on our biological natures. It is that it is only given our biological natures that this world exists *for us*, that we have access to the world in this mode.

One consequence of this is that different animals inhabit different perceptual worlds even though they inhabit the same physical world. The sights, sounds, odors, and so on that are available to humans may be unavailable to some creatures, and likewise, there is much that we ourselves cannot perceive. We lack the sensorimotor tuning and the understanding to encounter those qualities. The qualities themselves are not subjective in the sense of being sensations. We don't bring them into existence. But only a very special kind of creature has the biological capacity, as it were, to *enact* them.[6]

4.9 Novel Colors?

If color experience is determined by laws of sensorimotor dependence, then it may be possible to give rise to novel color experiences by experimentally manipulating patterns of sensorimotor dependence.

This possibility—which is now being actively investigated by Kevin O'Regan, James Clark, and Aline Bompas—is suggested in the work of Ivo Kohler (1951). He designed glasses with split lenses that were yellow on the right side of each lens and blue on the left side. As a result of this, looking off to the right made things look yellow, and looking off to the left made them look blue. After a period of adaptation, Kohler found that subjects reported no apparent difference in how things looked with respect to color, regardless of the direction of gaze. The brain, it seems, adapts to the novel circumstances, and crucially, it does so in a direction-of-eye-movement dependent way. When goggles are eventually removed, subjects report striking aftereffects. Now things on the right look bluish whereas things on the left look yellowish, despite the fact that one is not wearing lenses. The qualitative character of color experience, in these cases, would seem to be determined not by the intrinsic properties of light entering the eyes, or by the intrinsic character of the way this light stimulates the photoreceptors, but rather by the perceiver's expectations of sensory effects of movement.[7] This is a striking example of the insufficiency of mere stimulation to determine content. Experience requires stimulation *and* sensorimotor understanding.

In order to test these ideas, O'Regan, Clark, Bompas, and their colleagues have recently attempted, in the laboratory, to generate new color experiences by manipulating sensorimotor contingencies. Using eye-tracking computers and displays, they have designed artificial conditions in which the color of a perceived object on a monitor depends on the direction or location of eye movements, and in which the active engagement of the perceiver in a manual task changes perceived color. In one test, for example, the subject tries to follow a big square on a screen with a little square. The big square moves randomly. The little square is under the subject's control. Whenever the squares are on the right, they are red. Whenever they are on the left of the screen, they are green. Later, subjects are presented with grey squares, either on the left or right of the screen, and asked to judge whether the square is more reddish or greenish. They found that for several minutes after the adaptation task, subjects judged squares on the "red" side of the screen to be reddish, and vice versa. (These results are unpublished.)

Despite these preliminary, findings, there are reasons to be doubtful that these studies will eventually yield robust, *novel* colors. First, color qualities, like numbers, are structurally located. Colors or changes in color don't come piecemeal, but rather en masse. To get interesting sensorimotor-contingency induced changes in color experience, you need to create changes that affect systematic relationships. Isolated changes affecting a class of stimuli presented on a computer monitor are too modest, too local, to jog the system one way or the other. To be successful, one would need, in effect, to construct a virtual environment.

Second, movement-dependent sensorimotor contingencies are typically low-level, depending on the fine-grained detail of our eyes, neural systems, and so on. Changes to patterns of sensorimotor dependence that leave these low-level dependencies unchanged are unlikely to be great enough to make a difference to experience.

Third, as I stressed earlier in this chapter, colors are *environmental* phenomena, and color experience depends not only on movement-dependent but also on object-dependent sensorimotor contingencies. To manipulate color in an interesting way, therefore, one must manipulate the way object appearance interacts with conditions of illumination, colors of surrounding objects, and so on.

One way to see why the color studies of Bompas, O'Regan, and Clark are unlikely to work is that color, in humans, is too bound up with our broader sensorimotor and cognitive lives. Color experience is grounded in the complex tangle of our embodied existence. Chances for success might be better if one were to try to generate "color experiences" in a novel prosthetic system such as, for example, Peter Meijer's *The Voice* or Bach-y-Rita's TVSS. (I discuss *The Voice* briefly in section 4.10.) Perhaps we could define a color stimulus as one that varies under certain kinds of prosthetic "eye" movements and certain kinds of changes in environmental conditions. We can hypothesize, then, that by manipulating these conditions it would be possible to enable a form of primitive color experience in the blind.[8]

Perhaps the most serious problem confronting experimental work in this area is the problematic status of novel colors themselves. (See Thompson 1995 for an extended discussion.) Suppose that C is a novel color. Either C stands in relations of similarity to familiar colors along the three dimensions of hue, saturation, and brightness, or it does not. If it does, then C isn't really a *new* color. At best, it is a color that is brighter, or darker, or redder, say, than other arbitrarily chosen colors. Crucially, it occupies a position in our familiar color space.

Suppose C *does not* stand in these sorts of familiar relations to familiar colors, namely, it does not stand in relations of similarity or difference to known colors along the three dimensions of hue, saturation, and brightness. Then we can reasonably ask: What reason would we have for thinking that C is a color at all, and not, say, a sound or some other perceptual quality?

To discover a new color, then, one would have to discover a new color *system*, that is, a system of relations among qualities that is sufficiently like that holding among our colors as to count as a different *species* of color (as argued by Thompson 1995). We're in a domain here where there will be a

certain amount of arbitrariness (just as there is when it comes to individu-
ating species in biology). Compare number systems. From the standpoint
of the natural numbers, there couldn't be a number that was not, say, 0, or
the successor of 0, or the successor of some number that is the successor
of 0, and so on. What about 0.5? From the standpoint of the naturals, 0.5
just isn't a number. The rationals form a different and autonomous system,
one governed by different rules. It is reasonable to say, of this system, that
it is a *number* system, but surely nothing forces us to say this. (This is what
Wittgenstein had in mind when he said that the concept of number is a
family resemblance concept.) This doesn't mean that it's arbitrary whether,
say, imaginary numbers, or transfinite numbers, are really numbers. It isn't
arbitrary at all. But the rationality of these classifications reflects more
about our interests and classificatory aims than it does about the intrinsic
properties of naturals, transfinites, and so forth.

Could there be different, partially incommensurable color systems?
Could there be systems of relations among qualities that were *color-like*
even though the resulting "color" space was not at all like our own?

This is an empirical question, but it is one that, for the reasons given
previously, is very much wrapped up with conceptual and methodological issues. It's hard to see how there can be any straightforward resolution.

As a comparison, consider the question of whether two different biological perceptual systems are, in fact, visual. When the species are closely
related in evolutionary space, the question may be pretty straightforward.
But what about when we are considering cases of more remote lineages, for
example, perceptual systems in the primate, the bee, and the octopus? The
same issue confronts us when we consider sensory substitution systems,
which ground perceptual modalities in unusual systems. Is there a clear
fact of the matter about whether a system is a visual system?

In chapter 3 I proposed (building on work with O'Regan [O'Regan and
Noë 2001 a,b,c; Noë and O'Regan 2002] and with Hurley [Hurley and Noë
2003a; Noë and Hurley 2003]) that a system is *visual* if it is identical to our
visual system or suitably similar with respect to sensorimotor patterns (see
also Noë 2002a). In practice, this means that there will be a continuum of
cases. Creatures with bodies like ours would have systems that are visual in
the way ours are. Indeed, only such systems can participate in the identical range of sensorimotor interactions that we participate in. However, we

can grant that perceptual systems embodied very differently could also be visual, at least to some degree; what is decisive is the degree to which the embodiment allows for the relevant sensorimotor isomorphisms. If the enactive approach is right, even creatures with significant differences in their embodiment—even artificial systems—could see as we do, could enjoy perceptual experiences with visual content.

But there would be experiential differences between humans and creatures such as these. There would be ineliminable incommensurabilities between them and us. This indicates, I think, how we should approach the question of novel color systems.

To imagine a creature with a novel color space is precisely to imagine a creature who is perceptually aware of qualities whose natures are governed by (roughly) the kinds of movement-dependent and environmental laws of sensorimotor dependence typical of normal human color perception, but with differences. The perceived quality in question will count as color insofar as it has, at the right level of abstraction, the same general sort of sensorimotor profiles as our colors do.

4.10   Sounds and Other Qualities: The Account Extended

This account of color and color experience can be extended to other qualities perceptible in other sensory modalities. Here I give a brief outline of the way one might proceed in the case of sounds.

It is useful to remind ourselves that hearing, like sight and touch, is a way of learning about the world. You hear the car backfire. You hear that the car backfires, and that the car is, say, a block or so away in that direction. Auditory experience, like visual experience, can represent how things are, and it can also represent how things sound in relation to oneself. With this in mind, consider that the sensorimotor laws governing our auditory relation to things and events are strikingly different from those governing vision or touch. We continuously adjust our head in order to better take in noises belonging to one happening or another, and the fact that we do so shows that we are implicitly familiar with the way changes in our relation to events alters our sensory stimulation. The distinctively *heard* qualitative character of events is not determined by the intrinsic nature of the sensory stimulation, or by the fact that the stimulation sets up neural activity in the cochlea and auditory cortex. Rather, it is determined by the fact that the stimulation is governed by auditory sensorimotor laws. As evidence for this claim, consider the recent development of Peter Meijer's *The Voice* auditory-visual substitution system. Visual information made available to a camera activates sounds that vary in their audible qualities (pitch, etc.). A long-term blind subject describes herself as seeing again after a period of training. The neural and mechanical basis of *The Voice* perception is not like that of vision, yet it gives rise to experiences with *visual* qualitative character (at least to some degree). It can do this because it is governed by vision-like sensorimotor regularities (O'Regan and Noë 2001a,b; Noë 2002a; Hurley and Noë 2003a,b).

Sounds are color-like, and sound perception is like color perception. The distinctive feature of color perception, as we have seen, is that colors (apparent and real) are a kind of appearance. Colors are visually salient ways objects affect their environment. Sounds, in comparison, are audibly salient ways in which events (see O'Callaghan 2002) affect their environment. When you hear the car backfire, what you hear is the way the event (the backfiring) affects the ambient acoustic array, that is, the way a medium-filled environment is structured by this sort of disturbance to the medium. To hear that the car is backfiring a block or so over there is thus to hear a disturbance and to understand, implicitly, that the sound of that disturbance would change as your spatial relation to the sound source changed.

There are constancy effects as well in the domain of hearing. The siren sounds louder as we approach it, even though we can also tell, by hearing, that it hasn't actually gotten louder. We hear it as louder thanks to the change in our relationship to it. Likewise, you can perceive that the person near you and the person over there are talking at about the same volume, even though the person nearer prevents you from hearing the one over there (the one drowns out the other, which is auditory occlusion). How things sound varies as one moves in relation to sound sources. The patterns of change as one moves make the world available to perception.

5   Perspective in Content

The stimulus, as we know, is of infinite ambiguity, and ambiguity as such . . . cannot be seen.
—Ernst Gombrich

The world we live in is the world of sense data; but the world we talk about is the world of physical objects.
—Ludwig Wittgenstein

5.1   A Duality of Content

What do we perceive? Part of what makes the study of perception so difficult is the fact that there is more than one way to characterize what we perceive accurately. On the one hand, we perceptually experience objects, events, and states of affairs. You see the deer crossing the road; you hear your friend doing the dishes in the next room; you touch the hairbrush. On the other hand, all we ever experience are those aspects of things that are visible, audible, and so forth: for example, how they look or sound or feel from here.

Perceptual content has a dual aspect. There's the way experience presents the world as being, as it were apart from your perspective. This is one aspect of its content. And there is *the way* the world is presented in experience, a way that always incorporates some reference to how things look or sound or feel from your vantage point. So, for example, your experience presents you with the circularity of the plate, but also with the elliptical shape it presents from here, with the color of the wall, and also the way it looks with respect to color across its surface from here, in this lighting.

The sense-datum theory, which descends from Hume's phenomenalism, insists that you aren't entitled to the more robust, world-referring content

(Ayer 1955; Price 1948, Hume [1739–1740] 1975). All you have in your experience—all your experience grants you—is appearance. Kant and the ordinary-language tradition of Austin (1962) and Ryle ([1949] 1990) are scornful of the philosophical naïveté that underwrites the sense-datum theory. They insist that, as Strawson (1979) might have put it, the only veridical way to characterize your experience as it is given to you is in terms of the way it presents the world to you as being (say, as an experience as of a deer).

The truth lies somewhere in the middle, as the discussions of earlier chapters suggest: The plate looks to be circular (it really does) *and* it looks elliptical from here (it really does). The wall looks to be uniform in color across its surface *and* it appears brighter, where it falls in direct light. A theory of perceptual content needs to acknowledge and account for this dual aspect of perceptual content.

The enactive view can do this. The key, developed in the accounts of perceptual content in chapters 3 and 4, is that perceptual experience is a way of encountering how things are, but it is a way of encountering how things are by making contact with how they appear to be. How they (merely) appear to be plus sensorimotor knowledge gives you things as they are. What prevents this "two-step" account from collapsing into the sense-datum position is the fact that there is no reason to think that appearances—how things look, sound, or feel—are sensations or mental items. How things look, for example, is precisely a feature of the way things are. Looks are genuine, relational properties of things. But looks are not relations between things and your mind; they are relations between objects and the environment in which you find yourself as a perceiver. How things look with respect to shape, for example, is a fact about the thing and a vantage point, a vantage point you may happen to occupy.

To summarize: Perceiving how things are is a mode of exploring how things appear. How they appear is, however, an aspect of how they are. To explore appearance is thus to explore the environment, the world. To discover how things are, from how they appear, is to discover an order or pattern in their appearances. The process of perceiving, of finding out how things are, is a process of meeting the world; it is an activity of skillful exploration.

5.2 The Discovery of Appearances

We see by seeing how things look. This claim might seem to fly in the face of the fact that most perceivers can barely describe the perspectival shapes and sizes of things around them. A sensitivity to phenomenology—to how we naturally think about our experience when we have it and take it at face value—might seem to require that we reject the idea that perceptual awareness is, in the first instance, an awareness of perspectival qualities.[1] Perceptual experience, so this line of thought goes, is *transparent* (as mentioned in section 2.9). To reflect on experience is to reflect on the world as it is given in the experience.

In what sense are we really aware of perspectival properties? Are you aware, when you see the chair, of its perspectival shape and size? Gombrich (1960–1961) gives a suggestive example: Stand before the fogged up mirror in your bathroom after showering. Outline your head in the mirror with your finger. You will be astonished at how small the visual image of your head is. But this is the perspectival size of your head as seen in a mirror. Do we really want to say that whenever you see yourself in a mirror, you also see your head as having this occlusion size?

We may be in the vincinity here of a genuine indeterminacy in experience. Is there a fact of the matter, we might ask, about how the plate *really* looks? Does it really look elliptical? Or really look circular? The answer ought to be: There is a sense in which how things look depends on what you are interested in, or on what you ask, on how you probe. There is a sense in which there is no thought or interest-neutral fact of the matter about how things look. It's relative. What is *not* relative, though, is the fact that one and the same experience of the plate must contain within it the possibility of (at least) these two readings. You must be able to shift between these different ways of thinking about your perceptual relation to the plate.

Perception is a way of finding out how things are from an exploration of how they appear. In this sense, appearances are perceptually basic. As I argued in chapter 3, this is the truth in the sense-datum theory. Our acceptance of this in no way commits us to the idea that, as it were, our perceptual consciousness is confined to sense data. This is so because appearances are not merely sense data; they are aspects of how things are. Perception is an activity of learning about the world by exploring it. In that sense, then, perception is mediated by appearance. Our account of perceptual content must acknowledge this.

There can be little doubt that we do not normally reflect on apparent shapes, sizes, and colors when we look around. Our attention is typically directed elsewhere, to how things are in this or that respect. But this does not imply that we are not sensitive perceptually precisely to how things appear. Consider that normal perceivers are in fact quick to acknowledge, with almost no prompting, that there is a sense in which the circular plate looks elliptical (as well as round), or that the nearer tree looks larger than the farther one (even though one can tell they are of the same size by looking), or that objects change colors as lighting changes (even though of course they do not *actually* change color). This shows, I think, that perceivers are implicitly familiar with perspectival properties, and with the way they vary as we move about in the environment. It is true that Gombrich's mirror case is somewhat astonishing; but this may have less to do with perspectival properties than with the puzzling character of reflections. Strikingly, when as children we are first taught familiar "tricks" of perspectival drawing (e.g., how to produce simple 3-D effects, etc.), we have a striking "Aha!" experience, a feeling of satisfying recognition—something implicit was made explicit.

Sean Kelly and Hubert Dreyfus have criticized my position (in conversation) as phenomenologically wrongheaded. (See also Kelly, forthcoming.) There is no doubt, Kelly reasons, that we can detach ourselves from our familiar *engaged attitude* and take up the sort of detached attitude that enables us to direct our attention to perspectival properties of how things look. In the detached attitude, you can reflect on the merely elliptical perspectival shape of the plate. Kelly and Dreyfus insist that it is a mistake—Husserl's mistake?—to think that when you experience the round plate in the engaged attitude you also, at the same time, experience it as elliptical. Similar points are made by Kelly about color constancy. (See chapter 4, note 2.) You can see the wall as uniform in color, and as variable in color as a result of differences in the way it is illuminated, but you can't see it both ways at the same time.

This seems exactly wrong to me. When you look at the wall, you see its uniform color *in* its evident variation in color across its surface. When you look at a circular plate, held up at an angle, you experience its circularity *in* its merely elliptical shape.[2] When you look at a tomato, you experience it as full-bodied and three-dimensional even though you don't see its sides or back; you experience its three-dimensionality in its visible parts. Part of what makes the study of perception so difficult is the necessity of acknowledging not only this dual aspect in perceptual content, but the prima facie conflict in perceptual content. The enactive view—as laid out in this book—seeks to take this problem seriously.

There is a sense in which we move about in a sea of perspectival properties and are aware of them (usually without thought or notice) whenever we are perceptually conscious. Indeed, to be perceptually conscious is to be aware of them. This is perhaps what Wittgenstein had in mind in the epigraph at the outset of this chapter. Perhaps also it is a recognition of this fact that led Ruskin ([1856] 1971), on behalf of Impressionism, to claim that painting requires the *discovery* of visual appearances.

It is also important to underscore that to turn our attention to perspectival aspects of our perceptual content is no less to turn our attention to the world, and so it is, no less, to think of experience as transparent. In both cases, we turn our attention to the world, but the world thought of in different ways. We are used to thinking about the world we perceive not as a domain for perceptual activity, but as consisting of or containing the properties and facts that interest us. The fact that we rarely pay attention to the world *as a domain of perceptual activity* does not count against the claim that we inhabit it as such. To understand perception, it is necessary to bring into focus the fact that the world we inhabit and explore as perceivers is encountered in the first instance not as housing those facts and properties, but rather (in Adrian Cussins's phrase) as *mediating* our active exploration (Cussins 2003). The world as housing the facts and properties of interest to us is encountered due to our practical grip on the world as mediating or as affording perceptual activity. In this sense, we perceive the world by perceiving how the world merely appears, what it affords us.

It's worth reiterating that the claim that we experience perspectival properties is not meant to challenge the rival claim that we experience things as they are. For crucially, the encounter with the world *as it presents itself to us* is precisely the way we make contact with how things are apart from how they perceptibly appear to us to be.

5.3   Two Aspects of Content

Perceptual content—what philosophers call representational content, or *how* the experience presents the world as being—is two-dimensional. It can vary along a *factual* dimension, in regard to how things *are*. And it can vary along a *perspectival* dimension, in regard to how things *look* (or appear) from the vantage point of the perceiver. Visual experience always has both these dimensions of content.[3] This corresponds to the fact that perception is, at once, a way of keeping track of how things are, and also of our relation to the world. Perception is thus world-directed and self-directed.

Now there is no general requirement that for an experience to be veridical, it must be completely veridical. You can succeed in seeing a spoon, for example, even if the spoon nonveridically looks bent (say, because it is in water). And so, likewise, there is no hard requirement that for a perceptual experience to be veridical, it must be veridical along both dimensions of its content. We frequently enjoy visual experiences that are perspectivally nonveridical but factually veridical. This is the case, for example, when you spy on someone while underwater using a periscope. The experiences you have with the periscope represent how things are, but they *mis*represent your relation to how things are—that is, they misrepresent the perspectival content of your experience.[4] When you watch a live sporting event on television, you are able to track what's happening, but you do so in a perspectivally nonveridical way. Perhaps you adopt the standpoint of one or more cameras. Crucially, you don't correctly or veridically experience the event's spatial relation to yourself. It would be dogmatic to deny that you genuinely *see* the sporting event, that you see it "through" or by means of the television cameras. But it would be just as dogmatic to insist that there is no difference whatsoever between normal perception, in the here and now, and televisual perception. The difference is one that is now easy to explain: When you witness events in person, your experiences track not only how things are, but also how things are in relation to you.[5]

For an experience to be veridical simpliciter, then, is for it to be veridical along both factual and perspectival dimensions. But I have already drawn attention to the fact that veridicality is not sufficient for perception. Just as there are two dimensions along which an experience can be veridical, so there are two dimensions along which it can be *veridically hallucinatory*. Things can turn out to be the way they seem, even though their seeming that way is independent of the fact that they are that way, and they can turn out to stand in the relation to you in which they seem to stand, even though your relation to how things are has no effect on how they seem.

For an experience to be not merely veridical (simpliciter), but genuinely *perceptual* (simpliciter and, as we might put it, normal), the right sort of counterfactual supporting dependence must be maintained along *both* dimensions of content. It is pretty clear what that requires as far as factual content is concerned: that things would have looked different had they been different. But what does it require as far as perspectival content is concerned? The answer is at hand: It requires that had one's relation to how things are been different, things would have looked different (even if how things in themselves are were unchanged). It requires, therefore, that how things look depends, in a fine-grained, closely coupled sort of way, on movements. We need a further movement-dependence requirement to the effect that how things look depends (in a counterfactual supporting way) on movements (of the relevant type).

When you take your experience at face value, you encounter it as raising questions not only about how things are, but about how we stand in relation to how things are. To be a perceiver, then, you must understand, implicitly, that your perceptual content varies as things around you change, and that it varies in different ways as you move in relation to things around you.

5.4 Causation in Perception

Philosophers have tended to deploy a somewhat too narrow conception of perceptual (that is to say, *representational*) content. We have considered one instance of this already (in chapters 3 and 4), namely, the assumption that perceptual qualities such as perspectival shapes, sizes, and colors must be thought of as properties not of the experienced world, but rather as properties of the experiences. Against this, I have proposed that these are genuine properties capable of being captured in experience. In this chapter, so far, I have sought to make explicit what this more inclusive conception of perceptual content requires: It requires the recognition that perception is a way of encountering not only how things are, but how things are *in relation to* the perceiver. Perceptual experience is intrinsically perceiver-centered:

Visual experience is always experience of things being some way or other *from a point of view*. Perceptual content has an intrinsically perspectival aspect.

This is the key, it turns out, to making sense of an enduring philosophical puzzle concerning the question whether perception is a *causal* concept.

According to Grice's original proposal (1961), S sees that o is F if and only if S has a visual experience as of o's being F; o is F; and o's experience depends, causally, on o's being F. The point of the causal-dependence clause is to rule out what came, later on, to be known as veridical hallucination—namely, cases in which one enjoys a veridical visual experience that nevertheless falls short of being genuinely perceptual (Lewis 1980). Grice's example went like this: Suppose there is a clock on the shelf and that you have a veridical experience as of its being there. But suppose that the cause of your experience is not the clock's being on the shelf, but, say, posthypnotic suggestion. In such a case, you do not succeed in seeing that the clock is on the shelf, even though your experience is veridical. What explains this failure, so Grice proposed, is the fact that in this case the requirement of causal dependence is not met.

Grice was clearly on to something. Perception *is* a causal concept. But it quickly became clear (to Grice as well) that the causal theory was too weak, and that reasonable efforts to strengthen it were likely to make it too strong. Suppose that what produces your experience as of the clock on the shelf is a manipulative neurosurgeon. Suppose further that this neurosurgeon makes it look to you as if there is a clock on the shelf *because* there is a clock on the shelf. In this case, your experience does satisfy the causal-dependence clause, but it does so in the wrong sort of way. The standard move is to strengthen the theory by constraining what counts as the right sort of causal dependence (e.g., Strawson 1974). The idea, roughly, is that for an experience to count as an instance of perception, it must depend on what it is as of in the normal way that perceptual experiences depend on what they are as of. Whatever else is true, it seems clear that the dependence mediated by the neurosurgeon's intentions is not normal.

Sadly, the strengthened causal theory faces two problems. First, it makes the philosophical analysis of perception beholden to empirical findings about what the correct causal relation is. This isn't such a big deal in our post-Putnamian intellectual climate; it may even be a virtue that the theory makes room for developing empirical science. The second problem is more serious: The strengthened causal theory is way too strong; it rules out as nonperceptual any cases in which the dependence of experience on how things are is abnormal. But we don't want to rule out all such cases. We can certainly make sense of the possibility of wildly abnormal forms of prosthetic or artificial perception.[6]

In the face of these difficulties, most philosophers despaired of giving a coherent analysis of "the perceptual relation" and moved on to other problems. I am no fan of the project of philosophical analysis: It's doubtful that there has ever been an analysis (i.e., a breakdown into necessary and sufficient conditions) of any philosophically interesting concept. But I do think that the causal theory is obviously right in certain ways, and it is obviously wrong in others, and it would be worthwhile to explain why this is so, even if we reject the project of analysis.

The enactive account of perception developed here enables us to do this. The problem with the causal theory is not that it fails to articulate with sufficient detail the right kind of causal relation, or that it relies on empirical rather than merely a priori considerations about what perception really is. The problem, rather, is that it relies on a much too simplistic account of the content of perceptual experience. Once we enrich our account of perceptual content, we'll get a better understanding of what's right in the causal theory, what's wrong, and how the causal theory needs to be amended to give a more illuminating account. Or so, at least, I argue.

The truth in the causal theory is this: It is a necessary condition on your seeing that such and such is the case not only that things are that way, and that you have a visual experience as of them being that way, but that you wouldn't have had that experience if they hadn't been that way. The causal theory captures the fact that perceptual experience—say, how things look—depends on how things are, and it does so in a way that supports the relevant counterfactual considerations.

A little reflection reveals that how things look does not *only* depend on how things are, and this is why the conditions mentioned in the previous paragraph are not jointly sufficient for genuine perception. There are aspects of perceptual content—aspects of how the experience presents things as being—that are not determined by how things are alone, but that depend, in addition, on the perceiver's relation to how things are.

Perception is a way of keeping track of how things are, but it is also a way of keeping track of one's relation to how things are (Hurley 1998; Noë 2002a). This point has two aspects. First, we experience not only how things are, but also how they look from here. We experience that the plate is round and that it looks elliptical from here. Its elliptical look from here is a genuine property of the plate—we see the shape and we see the perspectival shape from here—but it is also a relational property, one that depends on where "here" is. If we count perspectival properties (such as the elliptical look) as belonging to the representational content of experience (Harman 1990; Noë 2002a), then we are implicitly counting ourselves (or at least our vantage points or bodily locations) among those contents. Second, it is hard to understand how we could keep track of how things are if we were not also capable of keeping track of the ways in which our perceptual experience depends on what we do. The perspectival shape of the plate changes as we move. Indeed, as I have argued, our practical grasp on the way it changes as we move is precisely the way we succeed in experiencing its roundness. More generally, how things look (what one sees) changes with every movement of the eye or turn of the head.

Here's the crux: These *perspectival* aspects of perceptual content are only partly determined by how things are. They depend further on one's relation to how things are. Any account of perception that ignores this dependence of how things look on one's movements (i.e., on changes in one's relation to how things are), and that in effect ignores the distinctively perspectival aspects of perceptual content, will fail to provide an adequate account of what perception is. This is the problem with the causal theory.

Consider again problem cases such as that of the manipulative neurosurgeon. The way the case was initially described, it was reasonable to suppose that although factual dependence is preserved (it wouldn't have looked as if there were a clock on the shelf if there hadn't been one there), perspectival dependence fails. Perspectival dependence fails because it is natural to assume, given the way the case is described, that how things look wouldn't depend, in a nuanced and fine-grained way, on your movements and changing relation to how things are. How, after all, could the neurosurgeon preserve that kind of dependence? It's hard to imagine. Wouldn't the electrodes impede movement? So we naturally assume that, in a case such as this, head movements and eye movements make no difference to what is seen.[7] But this is just to say that dependence along the perspectival dimension fails and that the experience is, at least on this dimension, not genuinely perceptual. An experience that is unchanged as the eyes and head move, as the relation to the environment alters, is not *visual*, whatever else it is.

If this diagnosis of our inclination to view the manipulative neurosurgeon case as falling short of bona fide perception is along the right lines, then it ought to be possible to construct cases that do rise to genuine perception but that are equally deviant in their causal chains. Consider an example. An angel hovers near and makes it the case that your experiences depend, in a counterfactual supporting way, on how things are and on what you do. It looks to you as if there is a clock on the shelf, only because there is one there. And for every little twitch of your eye, there is a corresponding change in how things look. Moreover, the angel, let's say, is committed to maintaining these regularities come hell or high water. This is a way of seeing, I would say. It's an unnatural way of seeing, to be sure, but it's seeing nonetheless. And this would be so even if, as we might imagine, your visual cortex and retina are damaged so that, but for the angel's interventions, you would be blind. This would be a kind of divine prosthetic vision.

A second example is due to David Sanford (1997). Sanford asks us to imagine the case of "Chris-the-amazing-human-hearing-aid." Chris has superhuman powers of mimicry. She listens to sounds and conversations and is able to repeat them for you in a way that is qualitatively indistinguishable from the sounds themselves. Imagine that she is able to perform this feat in real time. According to Sanford, when you use a normal hearing aid to hear the people across the table, it is truly those people you are thus enabled to hear. But when you employ Chris-the-amazing-human-hearing-aid, it is actually Chris, and not the people across the table, that you hear. Chris does not, in other words, provide prosthetic hearing, even though, subjectively speaking, the experiences of using Chris and a top-notch hearing aid are indistinguishable. Counterfactually, Sanford is quick to reassure, Chris and the mechanical hearing aid are exactly on a par.

But this is not quite right. Sanford is mistaken when he claims that Chris and the authentic hearing aid are on a par as far as counterfactual dependence goes. They are only on a par as far as factual content is concerned. To appreciate this, consider that, as the case is described, it is natural to suppose that there is no dependence (of a counterfactual supporting sort) between how things sound (to you, the user of Chris-the-human-hearing-aid) and your spatial relation, say, to the people across the table. The relation of your body (and your ears) to the people across the table makes no difference to what you hear, so long as Chris is able to speak into your ears. With normal hearing, in contrast, or when you use a conventional hearing aid, this counterfactual supporting dependence is in evidence. Normally, that is, your auditory experiences of the people across the table will change if, for example, you turn away, or you get up and walk across the room. I propose, then, that the basis of the judgment that Chris does not provide a means of genuine prosthetic perception—a judgment that I think is right—is the fact that in this case how things sound depends not on your spatial relation to the object of hearing, but only on your spatial relation to Chris. You hear the sounds as they are heard by Chris. But to hear how they sound from her vantage point is not to hear how they sound (or how they would sound) from your own vantage point. It is, in short, the tacit presupposition of the violation of the principle of the dependence of experience on perspective and movement that explains the strength of the intuition that Chris doesn't enable genuine prosthetic hearing. Importantly, the fact of Chris's own agency, or the fact that it is she who is the object of hearing (and not the people across the table), makes no difference to the relevant facts of the case.

Suppose that Chris learns to produce the sounds that you would hear exactly as you would hear them if your ears were not defective. She produces the sounds in a way that is modulated to account for your movements and shifting spatial relation to the sound source and also in such a way as to account for ambient conditions. With Chris's assistance, you now hear exactly what you would hear if your ears were normal and in such a way that both the factual and perspectival content of the resulting experiences are genuinely perceptual. I think it is clear that Chris now enables prosthetic hearing (even though she is an agent with a mind of her own, and even though you hear the people across the room *by way* of hearing her voice). This becomes much more intuitively acceptable if we imagine that Chris is very small, so small that she can fit snugly in the ear. Chris is now causally responsible for its being the case that you have auditory experiences that depend, counterfactually, on what is going on around you *and* on your relation to what is going on. Chris-dependent hearing is full-fledged prosthetic perception.

The problem with the causal theory is not that it can't specify or constrain the causal relation. As the examples of divine prosthetic perception and Chris-the-human-hearing-aid show, no causal relation is so strange or unnatural that it is incompatible with genuine perception.[8] The problem is that the standard hard cases are underdescribed. They are presented in such a way that they leave the full content of the experiences unspecified, and so leave the sense that perspectival content is unaccounted for. This is what explains our judgment that cases such as that of the manipulative surgeon are not bona fide cases of perception. Crucially, it never had to do with causation, but with a failure to acknowledge the perspectival content of perceptual experience, and with a failure to recognize that perception is answerable not only to how things are, but to what we do.

The problem with the causal theory, its failing, is that it tended to rely on an account of perception restricted, as it were, to factual content alone. The causal theory leaves no room for perspectival content, and so for the role of *action in perception*.

5.5   Phenomenology, Art, and the Transparency of Experience

The transparency, or diaphanousness, of experience poses a problem for the theory of perception. To describe sensory experience, to reflect on it, is to turn one's attention *to* the experienced world. The experience itself is transparent. There's no experiencing it. There's only encountering the world—content—as you experience it. It would seem, then, that we cannot reflect on experience itself.

Can there be phenomenological reflection on experience? Can there be phenomenology? Can we make perception itself the object of our thought and awareness?

One way to appreciate the paradoxical nature of this problem is to consider it in connection with the problem faced by representational painting. If a painter sets him- or herself the goal of making a picture of a scene, and if this picture is meant to capture what the scene looks like, then the painter must attend not to the scene itself (as it were), but rather to the way the scene looks from here. The painter must consider the scene with an "unbiased eye" (Gombrich 1960–1961). As Ruskin writes: "The whole technical power of painting depends on our recovery of what may be called the *innocence of the eye*; that is to say, a sort of childish perception of these flat

stains of colour, merely as such, without consciousness of what they sig-
nify—as a blind man would see them if suddenly gifted with sight" ([1856]
1971, 27).

Ruskin is surely mistaken if he thinks that there is anything childish
about a skilled painter's perception of a scene. Strawson gets at this point
when he writes that it is wrong to hold, as the sense-datum theorist does,
that we "go beyond" our experience when we make perceptual judgments;
in fact, "we take a step back (in general) from our perceptual judgments in
framing accounts of our sensible experience" (1979, 46). To see the world
with an innocent eye is really, then, to view it with great sophistication,
stepping back from the way we naturally view it when we take our experience at face value. It is precisely what is distinctive of childish efforts to
draw a scene that it usually consists in a kind of picture-list of stereo-
types relying not on experience of how things present themselves visually,
but on knowledge of how things are (cf. Gombrich 1960–1961). So, for
example, the child makes grass green, even if he or she is depicting it in a
situation in which it would look golden brown, and the car is made larger
than a man, even though the man is in the foreground and the car is a
good distance away.

The paradox consists in this: A successful depiction of how things *look*—
of the apparent shapes and sizes and "stains of colour"—will necessarily be
a successful depiction of what is there, of how things are, of the world as
it is *in itself*. The child, in contrast, draws what is there without regard to
how it appears, and thus fails, in a sense, to make a picture. So we cannot
capture experience itself in our experience or thought.

Cubism is an artistic movement that captures the enactive insight.
Paintings by Braque and Picasso in the Cubist period demand precisely
that you attend to the fact that an object affords a potential for movement
and, therefore, sensory experience. The item is revealed from all sides at
once, as it were. The visual and the thought are commingled in the picture.

The question of whether there can be a phenomenology of experience
is mirrored, then, in the question of whether there can be an art of
experience.[9]

From the standpoint developed in this book, it is clear that the task of
phenomenology, and of *experiential* art, ought to be not so much to depict
or represent or describe experience, but rather to catch experience in the act
of making the world available. Experience is a kind of activity, an activity

that acquires content, as we have seen, thanks to the perceiver's application of a kind of sensorimotor knowledge. The aim of experiential art and phenomenology ought to be, or could be (or maybe simply "is") to draw our attention to an activity that, by dint of the fact that we can perceive, we are very good at.

There has been a considerable amount of investigation of pictures, pictoriality, and the relation between these and perception. A recurring theme in these discussions in the idea that a picture—say, a line drawing—depicts, because the drawing gives rise to a representation in us (e.g., the retinal image) like that which we would enjoy were we to look at the depicted scene. Pinker (1997) writes, for example, that a picture "is nothing but a more convenient way of arranging matter so that it projects a pattern identical to real objects." (1997, 216) The idea is that we experience the depicted scene, when we look at a picture, because the picture produces in us just the effect (or nearly the identical effect) that would be produced by the actual scene. As Pinker explains, "Whatever assumptions impel the brain to see the world as the world and not as smeared pigment will impel it to see the *painting* as the world and not as smeared pigment" (1997, 217).[10]

That the brain would need to make assumptions to get from the retinal image to a description of the world is clear: There's just not enough information in the retinal image to specify uniquely the environmental layout. Pinker enumerates some of the useful assumptions employed by the brain:

Surfaces are evenly colored and textured (that is, covered with regular grain, weave, or pockmarking), so a gradual change in the markings on a surface is caused by lighting and perspective. The world often contains parallel, symmetrical, regular, right-angled figures lying on the flat ground, which only *appear* to taper in tandem; the tapering is written off as an effect of perspective. Objects have regular, compact silhouettes, so if Object A has a bite taken out that is filled by Object B, A is behind B; accidents don't happen in which a bulge in B fits flush into the bite in A. (1997, 217)

A striking feature of this sort of approach to the problem of pictoriality is that it explains the pictorial powers of pictures in terms of the pictorial power of the retinal image. Seeing pictures, on this sort of view, is like *seeing* a retinal image. It is vision at one remove.

A similar idea has been proposed by Hayes and Ross, building on the work of Marr. They suggest that line drawings represent because they correspond to psychologically real means of representation in the brain. As they write, "the line-drawing-description that the visual system calculates from an actual line drawing imaged on the retina would need to be very similar to the line drawing itself if the line drawing is to be readily interpreted by the visual system" (Hayes and Ross 1995, 344). That is, what explains the fact that the visual system readily interprets the line drawing as having the pictorial content it does have is the fact that the line drawing is like the brain's own drawing of the depicted scene.

There is clearly something right in these proposals. When you view a picture and view it not as a bit of canvas or paper or whatever, but as a picture with a content, then there is a sense in which you *see* that which is depicted by the picture. So there must be some similarity between the state you are in when you look at a picture of *x,* and the state you are in when you actually look at *x.*

For reasons implicit in the discussion of earlier chapters, however, I am skeptical of this general line of approach. Perception is not a process of constructing an internal representation, so it seems implausible that pictures depict by producing the sort of representation in us that the depicted scene would produce. (And there are differences between the experience of a scene and the experience of its picture.)

The enactive approach suggests a rather different conception of pictorial representation. Pictures construct partial environments. They actually contain perspectival properties such as apparent shapes and sizes, but they contain them *not* as projections from actual things, but as static elements. Pictures depict because they correspond to a reality of which, as perceivers, we have a sensorimotor grasp. Pictures are a very simple (in some senses of simple) kind of *virtual* space. What a picture and the depicted scene have in common is that they prompt us to draw on a common class of sensorimotor skills.[11]

This is not the place to pursue this idea further. Whether or not this is along the right lines, my reason for going into this here is to call attention to something rather different: Most writings on the importance of art for perception focus on pictures and paintings as *objects of perception*, and explore the way in which the perceptual process itself depends on pictorial representations (e.g., the retinal image). I would like to suggest a rather different point of contact between art and pictoriality, on the one hand, and perceptual experience, on the other. It is not pictures *as* objects of perception, that can teach us about perceiving; rather, it is *making pictures*—that is, the skillful construction of pictures—that can illuminate experience, or rather the making or *enacting* of experience. Picture making, like experience itself, is an activity. It is at once an activity of careful *looking to* the world, and an activity of reflection on *what you see* and *what you have to do to see.*

The painter does need to discover appearances, as the Impressionists thought. Great care is needed, though, if we are to comprehend what sort of discovery this is. To discover appearances is not to turn one's gaze inward, as it were, to sensation and subjectivity. Rather, it is to turn one's gaze outward, to the world, but to the world thought of in a rather special way. The painter attends to the world *not as a* domain of facts and properties, states of affairs, and so forth, but rather, to the world as a domain of skillful perceptual activity.

Picture making takes up the phenomenological stance on the world. For this reason, it is to the activity of picture making that phenomenology can turn for instruction about how to do phenomenology. And this is the key to the seeming paradox of perceptual transparency. Perceptual experience *is* transparent: To reflect on experience is, of necessity, to reflect on the world around us that we perceive. But there are two ways to do this. One way, we reflect on that world as a domain of facts and states of affairs. The other way, we reflect on the world as a domain for active exploration. The dual aspect of experience is mirrored, therefore, in two ways of thinking about the world. Phenomenology, then, aims at the second way.

This has two important implications. First, phenomenology isn't reflection, if we think of this as a kind of introspection. Second, to engage in phenomenology is, if the enactive view is right, to study the way in which perceptual experience—mere experience, if you like—acquires world-presenting content. For the world as a domain of facts is given to us thanks to the fact that we inhabit the world as a domain of activity.

6 Thought in Experience

Without sensibility no object would be given to us, without understanding no object would be thought. Thoughts without content are empty, intuitions without concepts are blind.

—Immanuel Kant

Understanding is akin to an ability.

—Ludwig Wittgenstein

6.1 Is Experience Conceptual?

To perceive is not merely to have sensory stimulation. It is to have sensory stimulation one understands. This Kantian idea forms one of the main themes of this book. For Kant, and for more recent writers who have been influenced by him (such as Sellars 1956 and McDowell 1994a), the basic form of understanding is conceptual. Perceptual experience presents the world as being this way or that; to have experience, therefore, one must be able to appreciate *how* the experience presents things as being (cf. Peacocke 1983). But this is just to say that one must have concepts of the presented features and states of affairs.

There can be little doubt, then, that *some* perceptual content is conceptual; only someone in possession of appropriate conceptual skills could have a perceptual experience with that content. It couldn't look to you as if the ballerina tripped if you didn't know what a ballerina is, or what tripping is, and it couldn't sound to you like a backfire if you didn't know what a backfire is. Now there's knowing what a backfire is ("trucks, you know, they go bang sometimes, that's a backfire") and *knowing* what a backfire is ("a backfire is an explosion resulting from an air leak in the exhaust

system"). The fact that there are different standards for concept possession doesn't alter the fact that some perceptual content is framed precisely
in terms of what perceivers know about their worlds.

Is all perceptual content conceptual in this way? This is a more controversial question. In the last few years a growing number of philosophers
have been inclined to answer this question negatively; some content is
*non*conceptual. For example, it can look to an animal as if there is a flat,
greyish surface so many degrees to the right of center, even if the creature
does not have the concepts of "degrees," or "right of center," and so forth.
The experience can genuinely present the world as being that way for the
animal even though the animal has no cognitive apparatus for appreciating
how the experience presents the world as being.

At root, the basic impetus behind this idea that there is nonconceptual
perceptual content is the concern that to suppose that all perceptual content *is* conceptual is to *overintellectualize* perceptual experience (Hurley
2001). Concepts, so the worry runs, are, as Kant put it, predicates of possible judgment ([1781–1787] 1929, A69/B94). To have a concept is to be able
to make judgments. Judgments are made for *reasons*, and they aim at the
truth (Frege [1918–1919] 1984; Cussins 2003). To understand truth, you
must grasp (however implicitly) the *laws of truth* (i.e., logic), and you must
grasp the distinction between how things really are and how they merely
seem to be (Davidson 1982). Davidson has gone so far as to say that only
creatures with language can have truth-evaluable thoughts or possess concepts. To be a concept-user, then, is to be able to do all this. But—so the
concern goes—there are no such stringent, intellectual demands on being
a mere perceiver. After all, nonhuman, nonlinguistic animals can perceive,
and they clearly do not participate in the complicated intellectual practices
just adumbrated.

There are two persistent lines of argument for the view that the thesis
that all perceptual content is conceptual overintellectualizes the mind.
First, there is the basic line of thought just considered: Animals and babies
can perceive, but they don't have concepts; therefore, you don't need to
have concepts to perceive. Second, there is an argument based on the difference between perception and judgment (Evans 1982; Crane 1992).
Perceptual experience is not a kind of judgment, nor is it judgment-
dependent—that is, you don't need to judge that *p* to have a perceptual
experience as of *p*. But concepts are creatures of judgments, that is, as Kant

said, they are in nature just predicates of possible judgment; therefore, you don't need concepts to have perceptual experience.

I critically assess these arguments in sections 6.2 and 6.3. For reasons explained there, I don't find them very persuasive.

There is a third general argument against the conceptuality of perceptual experience: The representational content of experience (how the experience presents things as being) cannot be thoroughly conceptual, because, bluntly stated, we do not have concepts of all the things we can perceive (Evans 1982; Heck 2000; Peacocke 2001). That we do not, so it is suggested, is just a brute fact. For example, we don't have concepts of every shade of color we can see. Experience, as it is put, is more fine-grained than that.

There is obviously a sense in which this fineness-of-grain point is right. We have concepts of, for example, hue *categories*, but we don't have individual concepts (just as we don't have individual names) for *every* perceptible shade of color falling within a category. Likewise, when you see a person's face, for example, you encounter a range of shapes and colors and textures. You can hardly be said to have conceptual knowledge of each of these perceptible features. Nevertheless, in having perceptual experience, you encounter the world as *having* all those features. So there must, then, be nonconceptual content, that is, there must be ways experience presents the world as being of which perceivers lack the concepts.

Does this conclusion follow? This depends, not surprisingly, on what we mean by "concepts" and "conceptual knowledge."

As stated at the beginning of this chapter, one of the main themes of this book has been that to perceive you must have sensory stimulation *that you understand*. But unlike Kant and the tradition spawned by him, the form of understanding I have taken as basic is *sensorimotor* understanding. Mere sensory stimulation *becomes* experience with world-presenting content *thanks to* the perceiver's possession of sensorimotor skills.

In this chapter I propose that we should think of sensorimotor skills as themselves conceptual, or "proto-conceptual" skills.[1] Sensorimotor skills can play much of the role that concepts have been called on to play in Kantian theories of perceptual experience (such as McDowell's). And it is because of our possession of them that we can have experience with world-presenting content. Moreover, they can perform this role without facing the objections that have dogged the appeal to concepts in accounts of perception. For example, sensorimotor "concepts" are obviously the sort of skill that nonlinguistic animals and infants can possess, so the argument from animals gains no ground. In addition, sensorimotor concepts are cognitively basic; it may be that we can give an account of them as natural, and as at the basis of our normative, concept-using practices. I return to this later in the chapter.

Peacocke (2001) writes that "in characterizing the fine-grained content of experience, we need the notion of the experience representing things or events or places or times, given in a certain way, as having certain properties or as standing in certain relations, also as given in a certain way" (241). That is, he says, "We must, in describing the fine-grained phenomenology, make use of the notion of the *way* in which some property or relation is given in the experience" (240, emphasis in original). This is exactly right, and the distinction thereby indicated corresponds to the difference between factual and perspectival content drawn in the last chapter (and anticipated in the account of perspectival properties in chapters 3 and 4). Peacocke thinks we need the notion of nonconceptual content to characterize *ways* things are given in experience as distinct from the mere fact that a property or feature is given. It is the burden of this chapter, and this book, that we can *comprehend* the ways things are given in sensorimotor terms. The basis of our ability to experience things as given this way or that is sensorimotor. In fact, it is our ability thus to grasp things as given in sensorimotor terms that is the basis of not only our ability to experience them as given this way or that, but also our ability to represent the properties that are thus given.

If sensorimotor skills are a kind of simple concept, then perceptual experience depends on conceptual understanding, albeit of a special and primitive sort. Whatever one says here, it seems clear that many of the arguments for the nonconceptual character of experience are unsatisfactory (in interesting ways). This is my topic in the next four sections.

6.2 The Argument from Animals and Infants

As mentioned earlier, one of the prominent arguments against the idea that perceptual experience is conceptual turns on the fact that animals and infants can perceive, but they lack the sort of conceptual skills the conceptuality thesis supposes are necessary for perception. If this is right, then it shows a way in which the conceptuality thesis falsely exalts and "over-intellectualizes" perceptual experience.

No doubt nonhuman animals and human infants enjoy perceptual experience. It is also probably true that they lack the sort of "richly normative conceptual and inferential capacities" possessed by adult humans (Hurley 1998, 136). It would seem to follow, then, that perceptual experience is nonconceptual. But this does not follow. For it is far from obvious that animals and infants lack conceptual and inferential skills altogether.

Hurley has argued that a hallmark of adult human conceptual skills is the ability to deploy concepts in a manner that is context-free and general (cf. Evans's "generality constraint," as discussed in Evans 1982). As she writes, "Someone with conceptual abilities who can judge that a banana is green and that a sofa is soft can also in principle judge that a banana is soft, that a sofa is green, that it is not the case all bananas are green, that if a banana is green then it is not soft, and so on" (Hurley 1998, 138). But it would seem that animal would-be conceptual capacities satisfy this "generality constraint," at least to some extent. For example, we ought, surely, to refuse to characterize a monkey as recognizing another monkey *as of high status* (something ethologists do regularly, e.g., Cheney and Seyfarth 1990), if the monkey's capacity thus to recognize status were not to generalize to other conspecifics encountered on other occasions. And similarly, we would take a lion's general unresponsiveness to the presence of a gazelle, or its stalking behavior in relation to tree stumps, as reasons (although perhaps inconclusive) to refrain from describing the lion as stalking a particular gazelle on a particular occasion. In short, to the extent that we view an animal as subject to what Hurley refers to as the constraints of normativity and holism—as flexibly responsive to its environment in ways constrained by intentions and primitive practical rationality—then to that extent we must admit that it possesses, to at least some degree, conceptual and inferential capacities that differ from our own only in degree.

One source, perhaps, of the desire to withhold "richly normative conceptual and inferential skills" from nonhuman animals and infants is our adherence to a much too exalted conception of our own conceptual skills. We think of concept possession on the model of the possession of concepts such as that of *square*, to possess which a thinker must know the criteria that govern (and justify) its application. But not all concepts are like this.

As Wittgenstein's (1953) considerations on rule following suggest, at the base of our conceptual practices are conceptual skills that do not fit this Socratic or Fregean model.[2] When I judge that something is red, for example, I do not do so on the basis of criteria. I can give no reason for my judgment that it is red other than the fact that, for example, I can see it. I judge an argument to be valid because I recognize it to be an instance of *modus ponens*. I do not then owe an explanation of what it is that makes modus ponens valid. That is, my grasp on validity does not in general require this. (This is true even if it is the case, as it is, that there are standpoints from which one can reasonably ask, *What makes a thing red?* (e.g., *what physical properties*), and *What makes modus ponens valid?* (e.g., *what metamathematical properties*). For crucially, one is not required to take up this sort of physical stance, or this sort of metamathematical stance, respectively, when deciding on the color of a thing, or in evaluating an argument's validity.)

The significance of this point is that our possession of such basic conceptual skills is strikingly situation-dependent and context-bound. We can tell by looking that a thing is red, or an argument valid, even if we cannot articulate the reasons why.[3] But this situation dependence and context boundedness are features that human conceptual and inferential skills seem to share with the much more primitive skills of animals.

In general, evidence that a particular animal cognitive skill is a "context-bound island of rationality" provides little support for the claim that animals lack conceptual skills altogether. Consider an example adduced by Hurley:

Sarah Boyson's chimp Sheba displays an island of instrumental rationality that does not generalize. Sheba was allowed to indicate either of two dishes of jellybeans, one containing more than the other. The rule was: the jellybeans in whichever dish Sheba indicated went to another chimp, and Sheba got the jellybeans in the other dish. Sheba always chose the dish containing more jellybeans, even though this resulted in her getting fewer. Despite her apparent frustration, she seemed unable to indicate the smaller amount in order to get the larger amount. Boyson next substituted numerals in the dishes for actual jellybeans. She had previously taught Sheba to recognize and use the numerals '1' through '4'. Immediately, Sheba began to choose the smaller numeral, thereby acquiring the correspondingly larger number of jellybeans for herself. The substitution of numerals seemed at once to free her to act in an instrumentally rational way, as she had been unable to when faced directly by the jellybeans. When the numerals were again replaced by jellybeans, Sheba reverted to choosing the larger number. (2001, 426–427)

Does this case lend support to the idea that Sheba lacks the relevant quantitative concept? I think not. As described, the case would seem to show that Sheba, although lacking full-fledged inferential skills, has some partial grasp on what it is for one dish of jellybeans to have more than another. After all, she chooses the dish with the greater number of jelly-beans, because it has the greater number of jellybeans, and because she cannot help herself from reaching out for the greater number. (See Boyson et al. 1996.)

A second source of our unwillingness to admit that animals and infants possess primitive conceptual and inferential skills is that we hold to an oversimplified conception (a caricature really) of what it is to make use of a concept in thought and experience. We think of concepts as brought into play only in the context of what we might call *explicit deliberative judgment*. But conceptual skills can also enter thought as background conditions on the possession of further skills of one sort or another. For example, the monkey's possession of the concept of a kin-group member is exhibited, we might say, in its differential treatment of its relatives even when the monkey never engages in anything like explicit delibera-tive judgment that so-and-so is kin. This interpretation of the monkey's cognitive accomplishment is compatible with its being the case that the monkey may lack knowledge usually taken to be necessary for pos-session of kinship concepts (e.g., knowledge of the biological basis of kinship, etc.).

This way of thinking about concept possession suggests that concepts can enter into an experience not so much because they are judged, by the possessor of the concept, to apply, but because their possession is a con-dition on the having of that experience. We would not credit a person with the visual experience as of an anteater, if we did not believe the person has the concept *anteater*.[4] This would be so even if no deliberative judg-ment is made in the context of perception. From this standpoint we can agree with Hurley's thought that one can have reasons for acting even though one is not capable of appreciating reasons for forming beliefs about what should be done (i.e., even though one's practical reasons do not dis-play the inferential promiscuity of fully conceptualized reasons). This pos-sibility, however, does not show that the reasons in question lack conceptual content. For there is a way of bringing concepts to bear in thought and reasoning other than their deployment in deliberative judgment.

6.3   Experience Is Not Judgment

Kant held that concepts are predicates of possible judgment (Kant [1781–1787] 1929, A69/B94). The basic thing we do with concepts is apply them in judgment (i.e., we decide whether or not something falls under the concept in question). Given this, the claim that perceptual experience is conceptual has seemed to carry with it the danger of confusing perceiving with judging. The danger has been real; at least one excellent philosopher has held the view that to perceive that *p* is to come to form the belief or judgment that *p* (Armstrong 1968).

This is obviously wrong. It is not the case that things always look the way they are. Nor is it the case that, when one has a visual experience, say, one must be even *inclined* to judge things to be the way the experience presents them as being. Experience is belief-*in*dependent in precisely the sense that it can look to you, say, as if the two lines of the Müller-Lyer illusion differ in length, even when you have drawn them yourself and know them to be of the same length (Evans 1982, 123–124).

The fact that experience is belief-independent, however, does not undercut the conceptuality thesis, for the conceptuality thesis is not committed to the idea that perceptual experiences are judgings or believings. To undercut the conceptuality thesis one would need to demonstrate not belief independence, but belief in*difference*. To establish that, one would need to show that perceptual experiences are not even *relevant* to how one takes the world to be. But it is unlikely that that is something that can be shown.

The interest of the fact that the lines can look unequal even when one knows that they are not is precisely that, this divergence notwithstanding, experience continues to have a bearing on judgment. How things look to one remains at least relevant to how one *ought* to judge things to be. This is the crucial point. One cannot have the experience that *p* without at least recognizing—in some sense—that the experience raises the question of whether *p*. Surely the significance of the belief *in*dependence of perceptual experience is not that belief (or judgment) and experience have no systematic rational connection, but that, rather, one *can* have an experience that represents things as being one way and a belief that represents them as being a different way. That is, judgments and experiences can diverge and even contradict one another. But to say that they *can* be in conflict is to say that they *can* be in accord; and this would seem to show that they have the same sort of content. The content of perceptual experience is conceptual not in the sense that it *is* judged, but in the sense that it *can be* judged. Perceptual experience raises the question of whether things are as the experience presents them as being. To have an experience, and to take it at face value, is to be presented with a possible way things might be.

In this sense we can say that the content of perceptual experiences are what Frege [1879] 1980 called 'judgeable contents' (or 'thoughts' (Frege [1918–1919] 1984). In perception you "entertain" a judgeable content in the sense that the experience puts the question of whether the content holds into play. To have an experience is to be confronted with a possible way the world is. For this reason, the experiences themselves, although not judgments, are thoroughly *thoughtful*. Perception is a *way of thinking* about the world.

There is a principled reason for thinking that experience is thoughtful in this way; it is a basic fact about perceptual experience that it is *intentional* (in the philosophers' technical sense). That is, perceptual experience presents things as being thus and such. It has content. It is *directed* toward, it is *about* the world (Anscombe 1965; Searle 1983). It is difficult to understand how one could have an experience with a given intentional content without being in a position to understand that content, that is, to understand how the experience presents the world as possibly being (cf. Peacocke 1983). Insofar as perceptual experience is intentional, experience seems to be bound up with our broader capacities to *think about* and *understand* the world.

This is related to the question of whether experience is direct. In perception we can always ask whether things are as the experience presents them as being. But we cannot raise the question, How does experience present things as being? Experience is constituted by its content (at least in part), and its content is always at least *as of* the world.

To summarize, one reason to think that perceptual experience is conceptual is that experience presents things to one as being this way or that; one needs an understanding of the ways experience is presented as being. The possibility that perceptual experience is conceptual in this way, however, does not entail that perceptual experience is belief-*de*pendent, and it does not carry in its wake an unreasonable assimilation of experience and judgment. All it requires is that we recognize that the content of experience, and the content of thought, can be the same.

6.4   Do We Have Concepts of Everything We Can See?

One of the most compelling lines of argument against the conceptuality thesis, and for nonconceptual content, starts with the fineness-of-grain considerations briefly described in section 6.1. These thoughts were first suggested by Evans, who wrote: "No account of what it is to be in a nonconceptual informational state can be given in terms of dispositions to exercise concepts unless those concepts are assumed to be endlessly fine-grained; and does this make sense? Do we really understand the proposal that we have as many colour concepts as there are shades of colour that we can sensibly determine?" (1982, 229). Evans's suggestion is that we don't have concepts of all the things we can see, that experience is more fine-grained than is our thought about experience. The wealth of perceptual experience outstrips what we can capture in thought. This point has also been argued with great force by Peacocke (1992, 2001).

Now, as indicated in section 6.1, it is certainly true, in one sense, that we don't have concepts of all the shades we can perceive: We don't have concepts of them in the way that we have concepts of, say, hue categories. This is reflected, as mentioned earlier, in the fact that we have names for hue categories (red, yellow, blue, green), but not for all the different determinate instances falling within each category. Is this fact an obstacle to the claim, advanced by McDowell, that one is "equipped to embrace shades of colour within one's conceptual thinking" (1994a, 56), and indeed that one is able to do so "with the very same determinateness with which they are presented in one's visual experience"?

I think we should answer this question negatively. In the next section I offer considerations in support of this conclusion. Before turning to this, however, I would like to consider two preliminary points that will help us understand what is at stake.

First, we should attend carefully to McDowell's choice of words in articulating the conceptuality thesis. He contends that "we are equipped to embrace all the shades we can see in conceptual thinking" (1994a, 56). He does *not* say that we are antecedently in possession of concepts (in the way we might be in possession of a vocabulary) of every perceptible feature (shade of color in this case). The claim that perceptual content is conceptual should not, then, be understood to amount to the claim that we have a kind of implicit mastery of a perceptual lexicon; it certainly needn't consist in the idea that we actually have names for everything. Instead we can think that what is required, if experience is to be conceptual, is that we are able to understand, or recognize, or appreciate, that the way our experience represents things as being is just that, *a way things might be.* Consider the visual experience of a face mentioned in section 6.1. I wrote that you can hardly be said to have conceptual knowledge of each of the face's perceptible features (e.g., the shapes and textures and colors). But is this true? Perhaps we could say that you do grasp these qualities, not in the abstract as it were (applying to each its proper name), but in the sense that you can think of them each as features a face might have, or as the ways a face looks. This would be a way of grasping what you see in thought.

Second, there is a tendency to mischaracterize the "richness" of perceptual content. Perceptual content may not be as rich as philosophers are tempted to suppose. Consider, for example, what Richard Heck has written about visual experience:

The leaves on the trees outside my window are fluttering back and forth, randomly, as it seems to me, as the wind passes over them.—Yet my experience of these things represents them far more precisely than that, far more distinctively, it would seem, than any characterization I could hope to formulate, for myself or for others, in terms of the concepts I presently possess. The problem is not lack of time, but lack of descriptive resources, that is, lack of the appropriate concepts. (2000, 489–490)

Is it really the case, as Heck writes, that our perceptual experience represents the details of the scene before me "far more precisely," "far more distinctively" "than any characterization I could hope to formulate"?

There are empirical considerations, reviewed in chapter 2, that call this into question. The phenomena of *change blindness* (O'Regan, Rensink, and Clark 1996, 1999; Rensink, O'Regan, and Clark 1997, 2000; Simons and Levin 1998), and *inattentional blindness* (Mack and Rock 1998) suggests that the content of our experience may, in important respects, be much less detailed and determinate than Heck's description would suggest. In particular, there is now good reason to believe that there is a surprisingly vast range of ways the scene around you could have been visibly different from the way it actually is, without any of these visible changes making a difference to the character of your experience. Imagine that every time you blink, someone (an evil manipulator) effects changes in the arrangements of papers on your desk, or books on your shelf, or chairs in your room, or leaves outside your window. Work on change blindness shows that if this were to happen, you might fail to notice, even though the changes are such that, if your attention were drawn to them, you would be shocked that you could have missed them. The upshot of this empirical work is that there is a sense in which you do not actually experience and monitor all the present detail. You do not really see it all. The actual content of your experience—of your attentive seeing at a moment in time—is much narrower and much sparser.

Phenomenological considerations also weigh against Heck's richness point. It is certainly true that we take ourselves to experience a detailed scene; but it is a mistake to suggest that we take ourselves to represent all the detail determinately in consciousness at a moment in time. My sense of the presence of the detailed world is grounded in my ability to gain access to that detail by the movements of my body or the shifts of my attention. The world is present to me now, not as represented, but as accessible. (This is a main theme of chapter 2.)

It would seem, then, that Heck's characterization of visual phenomenology is unreliable. He directs us to consider the fact that he is unable to characterize, either in words or in thought, the determinateness of the way the detailed world is given visually in experience, for example, the way "leaves on the trees outside my window are fluttering back and forth, randomly, as it seems to me, as the wind passes over them" (Heck 2000, 489). Heck takes this inability to show that experience outstrips our conceptual and linguistics resources. But there is another way to account for this inability. Perhaps what explains our inability to capture the detailed content of the experience in thought is that the experience does not determinately represent all that detail. It would seem that Heck's characterization of visual phenomenology is shaped by something like the Machian, snapshot conception considered, and rejected, in chapter 2.[5]

Heck has other ways of making the basic point that we lack concepts of all the features we can experience. For example, he writes (immediately before the passage quoted earlier): "Before me now, for example, are arranged various objects with various shapes and colors, of which, it might seem, I have no concept. My desk exhibits a whole host of shades of brown, for which I have no names. The speakers to the sides of my computer are not quite flat, but have curved faces; I could not begin to describe their shape in anything like adequate terms" (Heck 2000, 489). The thought here is that we don't have names, and so, it seems, we don't have descriptive or conceptual resources, to capture, in thought, even the simple qualities we can visually perceive.

I am not persuaded by these considerations. We must keep in mind the significance of the fact, discussed in chapter 4, that perceptual content is, as I put it there, *virtual all the way in*. There is no quality that is so simple that it is ever given to us all at once, completely and fully. However simple the object of our attention, the field of experience will outstrip what can be taken in at once. For this reason, no perceptual field is so simple as to be immune to change blindness. The upshot of this is that *all* detail is present in experience not as represented, but rather as accessible. One consequence of this is that when you do take your experience offline, as it were, and ask yourself *what is in my consciousness now*—that is, when you attempt to reflect on what is available in your current fixation—you will encounter an ineliminable indeterminacy; elements of the background, or the periphery of the visual field, or of present detail are present to perception *but indeterminately.*[6] The virtual character of perceptual content— a running theme in this book—explains the character and source of this indeterminacy. All the detail before me is *not* given in an instant; the sense of the presence of all of it is necessarily indeterminate insofar as it is grounded on the awareness that by looking here, or there, I can *determine* what I see. Given this, the explanation of the perceiver's inability to characterize what he or she experiences determinately is not the lack of the needed conceptual resources, but rather the fact that experience (thus taken offline) is really indeterminate. What considerations such as those advanced by Heck do not show is that the detail or quality of experience is given in a way that determinately outstrips what can be grasped in thought.

6.5 Embracing the World in Conceptual Thinking

With these considerations on the table, we are in a better position to see what is at stake in McDowell's conceptualist claim and to see how it can be defended. To have a perceptual experience is precisely to direct one's powers of thought to what one experiences; the experience, and the conceptualizing, are *one and the same* activity. Neither is logically or conceptual prior. As Kant held, concepts without intuitions are empty, intuitions without concepts are blind. The point here is exactly analogous to those made in earlier chapters on the necessity of sensorimotor knowledge: Mere sensory stimulation does not add up to experience. We don't *apply* sensorimotor knowledge *to* experience. Rather, we bring it to bear *in* experience; bringing it to bear in this way enables what would otherwise be mere sensory stimulation without world-presenting content *to be* experience. Perceptual experience *just is* a mode of skillful exploration of the world. The necessary skills are sensorimotor and conceptual.

We can begin to see how this account might be developed by considering again the fact that colors stand related to one another in such a way as to form a space or structure (similar points go for shapes and sizes). If one is familiar with the primitives of color—red, green, blue, yellow, black, and white—and if one understands that colors can vary on three continuous dimensions of hue, value, and intensity, it is possible, given one point in color space, to understand practically what is required to reach any other. It is true that for each shade we do not have a unique name. But the structural uniformities of color space make possible, as it were, the *conceptualization* of any given shade, for they make available the possibility of *color-concept-formulae*. One might speak of a shade of yellow-green similar to that of the such and such. Moreover, we can explain what we mean in a specific instance by reference to a specific visibly present shade. McDowell's basic idea seems to have been that perceptual demonstratives (e.g., "this shade," "that color") can be deployed to express demonstrative *concepts*—that is, concepts that are defined in terms of a perceptually present quality. It is by means of such concepts that we are able to "embrace shades of colour within one's conceptual thinking with the very same determinateness with which they are presented in one's visual experience" (McDowell 1994a, 56).

Such perceptual demonstrative concepts have given rise to Sorites worries. After all, one can't define "that shade" in terms of indiscriminability, in light of the familiar problem of the nontransitivity of indiscriminability. If x is indiscriminable from y and y is indiscriminable from z and z is not indiscriminable from x, then y is identical to two different shades (cf. Peacocke 1992, 83). But this is not a genuine Sorites problem, as

McDowell (1994a, 170–171) has argued. To see this consider Wittgenstein's remark (1953, sec. 50) that color samples should be regarded as instruments of language, as symbols. Samples are used to play a certain role as standards. They are deployed in explanations of meaning and are thus, in an important sense, not bearers of the property they are used to exemplify; qua sample, the sample of red is not itself red (although, for example, the card that is deployed as a sample ought to be). In this vein, Wittgenstein suggested that the standard meter was not itself one meter long. Surely the actual piece of platinum (or whatever) is one meter in length. Qua piece of metal its length is variable, depending on the conditions. But the length of the standard meter cannot vary; for insofar as the length of the stick in question does vary, it cannot perform its role as sample. Qua sample, it is not one meter long. It has no length. It is not an object of perception but a symbolic tool used for description. To be one meter is to be such that when the meter standard is laid against the thing, the edges line up.

And the same goes for color samples. When I explain a color term by reference to a sample, I am not saying of the sample that it is itself in the extension of the color concept I am defining. Anything that is the same as the sample (with respect to color) is in the extension. But then elements of the extension are not themselves, qua elements, and without further ado, suitable samples. And so the Sorites problem doesn't arise. In essence, since elements of the extension cannot be used as samples, the dubbing ceremony does not resemble the situation that engenders the Sorites worry. One says "this and anything like it (with respect to color) is red." One does *not* say "this and anything which is like anything which is like this (and so on ad infinitum) is red." The later formulation would lead to a Sorites problem, for it would treat each element of the extension as itself a suitable sample.

The key to understanding that we have the resources to embrace every shade we can see in conceptual thinking is to recognize that we have a kind of conceptual capacity that can be extended, as it were, *formulaically*, to every novel perceptual quality we encounter. Is this a reasonable proposal?

We are familiar with one domain of thinking in which we seem to possess precisely this sort of capacity: the domain of mathematics. Consider the following: We have concepts of *all* the natural numbers, even though there are infinitely many of them. How can our conceptual reach in this way extend to and "embrace" an infinity of objects? The answer may depend on the fact that numbers have structural features; they occupy positions in a space or system. To grasp the natural numbers, we do not need to have concepts of each of them antecedently, in storage, as it were, in a conceptual armory. It is enough that we can come up with the needed concepts when the occasion arises. We construct them to order, so to speak. Perhaps it would be better to say not that we need to construct *new* concepts for every number we can mathematically encounter, but rather that we need to be able to bring the novel number under our familiar concept, by extending the concept to embrace it.

We would not take seriously the argument that numerical thought is nonconceptual because it requires that we possess an infinity of number concepts or a concept of an infinity of different individual numbers. It is precisely the case that part of what is distinctive of mathematical thought is the fact that mathematical understanding enables us to "embrace numbers within our conceptual thinking" without having access to the prefabricated individual concepts of every number. What is distinctive about the concept of number may be precisely this formulaic aspect: that what falls under it flows from a rule. (This may have been what Wittgenstein meant, in *The Tractatus*, when he claimed (proposition 4.1272) that *number* is not a genuine concept, but merely a *formal* concept—that is to say, a variable with fixed logical syntax in the formalism. The idea was that anything that has the same logical-syntax of the variable *number* is a number, but that "_ is a number" is not a genuine predicate that ranges over a class of instances.)

Maybe colors, and other perceptible qualities, are like numbers. Maybe our grasp of color shares with number something like this formal or formulaic aspect. We understand the structural properties of color space in such a way that, for any given shade, we can embrace it in thought, even though we have never seen it before and so, in a sense, are not *re*-cognizing it. If this is right, then there is a sense in which there are no new experiences, no perceptible qualities requiring utterly new conceptual devices to comprehend them. In the same way, there are no new numbers. Properties of all numbers, and all experiential qualities, are given at once with the system.

One difference between numbers and colors concerns linguistic terms: We not only possess concepts of each of the natural numbers, we possess terms for each of them. The symbolism we use to represent numbers is such that it contains within it recursive procedures for generating number names ad infinitum. It is striking that we lack this sort of terminology for colors.

But this difference is only apparent. We *do* have a symbolism that is infinitely extensible in just this way. True, we don't have names for every perceptible shade, but we do have linguistic means for pinpointing any shade in color space, given a fixed starting point (a sample). So, for example, we can say, "No, this is not the red I want, I want something *lighter*, but not as light as this other sample." And so on.

A second difference between number and color concepts concerns re-identifiability. We may only construct needed individual number concepts when presented with the need to capture the individual in thought, but once we have done so, there are very strict criteria on what it is for something to *be* that number, and it is unproblematic to re-identify the number again in different circumstances. Colors are different. Perceptual demonstrative concepts may be such that we only grasp them when we are confronted with their instances, or, at the most, for a very short period of time thereafter (McDowell 1994a). If you show me a color sample and then show me a slightly different one the next day, I may not be able to tell that the second sample is different from the first. Does this show that I don't retain my grasp on the concept? Does this show that I never really had the concept? I don't think we need to accept this. To see why, consider a second analogy.

Some problems have the following feature: They are difficult to solve, but once you have a correct solution, it is easy to see that you've solved it. Take a jigsaw puzzle, for example. For any arbitrary piece, it's hard to give a general procedure for deciding where it goes. On the other hand, for most pieces, once you've placed it correctly, it's obvious that you have. This distinction is a hallmark of a certain class of computational problems that are known as nondeterministic polynomial (or NP) problems. An NP function (stated informally) is one that is easily checkable, once you've got a correct answer, but for which there is no general, relatively simple algorithm. A central theoretical problem in complexity theory is whether NP problems are all, in fact, feasibly decidable problems.

Consider the possibility that the question of whether a given perceptual demonstrative concept applies is, in effect, NP. These concepts are checkable: In the presence of their correct instances, it is obvious they apply. In their absence, however, it is difficult to know whether they apply.

If our concepts of colors are filled out with perceptual demonstrative concepts in this way, then it is not surprising that we are unable, as a general rule, to decide whether a given sample instantiates that concept. In particular, this fact doesn't show that we lack the concept in question. That's just not the way these concepts are used.

What *is* required is that we take seriously the question of whether a presented shade is or is not identical to the previously seen shade. The fact that we cannot tell doesn't show that there isn't a fact of the matter.

6.6   The Sensorimotor Grasp of Qualities

I propose that the kinds of perceptual concepts that are brought to bear in our experience of the shapes and colors and textures of daily life are, in effect, formal concepts in the way that numbers are formal. To comprehend a "new" number in thought is to extend a general concept to it thanks to our grasp of a general structure or framework or rule. As suggested earlier, in effect, there are no new numbers: *All of them* are given with the system. The claim is that this is how things stand with colors and shapes and textures and other perceptible qualities. In effect, there is no new experience. It's all familiar. There's nothing new under the sun. It is all comprehended by what we implicitly understand, by the structural spaces in which perspectival properties and apparent colors are located.

It is clear—more or less clear—what sort of grasp of mathematical principles enables us "to embrace" all natural numbers in conceptual thought. It is something like a grasp of the Peano axioms, or perhaps, the implicit grip on a Frege-style derivation of the Peano axioms from the Hume/Cantor principle of equinumerosity. But in what does our *generative* grasp on colors and shapes consist? It consists in our grasp (however fragile) of *sensorimotor* rules.

I have argued (in chapter 3) that the experience of shape depends on our implicit grasp of the way perspectival shape varies as we move in respect to an object. We don't have names for every aspect we encounter, but we have a grip on the way aspects vary. This grip is, in effect, our grasp of what it is for something to be *presented as* cubical, or spherical. It is much harder to make out what our grasp on the form of a shoulder, or a human jaw, or a hip consists in. But there is no reason, in principle, why it cannot consist in something very much like this. (See Koenderink 1984b for an attempt in this direction.) Similar kinds of considerations, as argued in chapter 4, go for color: Our grasp of color depends on our implicit mastery of the way appearances change as color critical conditions change.

I now propose that we consider these sensorimoter skills whose possession allows us to represent perceptual qualities in experience—to be conceptual (or proto-conceptual). Our possession of such skills enables us to embrace perceptual qualities in thought. This mastery provides a way of making what is new and hitherto unseen familiar and regimented. The proposal is that sensorimotor skills are the basis of our possession of the sort of recognitional capacities we draw on when we, as McDowell suggested, deploy perceptual demonstrative concepts to *make sense* of perceptual qualities. If this proposal is right, then we can understand how it is that we can bring a recognitional capacity to bear on something that we are seeing in fact for the very first time. And we can understand how we can genuinely be said to possess such capacities even though the range within which we can reliably and accurately apply them is very narrow indeed (i.e., only in the presence of an instance of the concept or for very short durations after).

6.7 Are Sensorimotor Skills Really Conceptual?

A basic concern about the conceptuality thesis is that it overintellectualizes experience. A main obstacle to offering a non-overintellectualizing account of the conceptuality of experience is an excessively demanding account of concept-using practices. As observed in section 6.2, we wrongly suppose that all concept use must take the form of explicit deliberative judgment, and that conceptual skills must rise to a level of acontextual generality. Understanding a concept may be much more like possessing a practical skill than we suppose. (This is how we should take Wittgenstein's idea that understanding is akin to an ability.)

Concepts are practical skills, and some practical skills—some sensorimotor skills—are simple concepts, or so I propose. Poincaré gives an example of the kind of considerations I have in mind:

Think, for example, of a sphere with one hemisphere blue and the other red; it first presents to us the blue hemisphere, then it so revolves as to present the red hemisphere. Now think of a spherical vase containing a blue liquid which becomes red in consequence of a chemical reaction. In both cases the sensation of red has replaced that of blue; our senses have experienced the same impressions which have succeeded each other in the same order, and yet these two changes are regarded by us as very different; the first is a displacement, the second a change of state. Why? Because in the first case it is sufficient for me to go around the sphere to place myself opposite the blue hemisphere and reestablish the original blue sensation. ([1905] 1958, 49)

The difference in the experience of the sphere's rotation and its actual change of color, Poincaré insists, does not consist in differences in the accompanying sensations. After all, there are no such differences. Rather, it consists in our implicit appreciation of the differences in the way sensations vary (or would vary) as a result of movement (on our part as well as that of the sphere). Poincaré suggests that this appreciation, or understanding, amounts to a grasp of the difference between an observed displacement and an observed change of state. The idea is amplified in this second example:

An object is displaced before my eye; its image was first formed at the center of the retina; then it is formed at the border; the old sensation was carried to me by a nerve fiber ending at the center of the retina; the new sensation is carried to me by *another* nerve fiber starting from the border of the retina; these two sensations are qualitatively different; otherwise, how could I distinguish them? Why then am I led to decide that these two sensations, qualitatively different, represent the same image, which has been displaced? It is because I *can follow the object with the eye* and by a displacement of the eye, voluntary and accompanied by muscular sensations, bring the image to the center of the retina and reestablish the primitive sensation. (Poincaré [1905] 1958, 49)

Here Poincaré explains that a visual experience can present an object as moving only when a perceiver has an implicit understanding of the way the perceptual relation to the object is mediated by distinct patterns of sensorimotor dependence. This is a central theme of this book (explored in detail in chapter 3). I want to suggest that the question of whether the perceiver is able, in experience, to represent the object's displacement is tantamount to the question of whether he or she possesses the relevant sensorimotor knowledge. But why not acknowledge that this sensorimotor knowledge constitutes the possession of the observational concept of displacement? The skills in which such concept possession consists would seem to be precisely sensorimotor skills.

One reason to refrain from granting that these sensorimotor skills make up our grasp of the relevant observational concepts is that the skills in question may be partially or wholly subpersonal. The patterns of stimulation of nerve fibers on the retina belong not to the perceiver's psychology but rather to the conditions that causally enable that psychology. Moreover, these patterns may occur below the threshold of consciousness.

I don't see why this fact—that at least some of the sensorimotor skills are subpersonal—should be taken decisively to weigh against the idea that these skills are conceptual. Their subpersonal character notwithstanding, the attribution of these skills is governed by the kinds of considerations of holism and normativity that characterize the domain of the conceptual. We would not credit a person with visual experience of an object's displacement unless further conditions of the following sort are met: Perceivers who can experience the object as visibly displaced will also expect that, say, the object will disappear from view if they shut their eyes, and they will be able to distinguish movements of the object from, say, movements of themselves relative to it. The possession of sensorimotor skills here amounts to the possession of the relevant observational concepts.

6.8   Context Dependence: A Reply to Kelly

Kelly (2001) proposes a different argument against the conceptualist thesis. He grants that the anti-conceptualist may not succeed in demonstrating that it is not the case that we have concepts of every quality we can experience. It remains true, however, he reasons, that there are ways in which experiences can differ that are at once representational (differences in how the experiences present the world as being), but that are not conceptual. He illustrates this with the phenomenon of color constancy: we may see that the wall is a uniform shade of white, say, despite the fact that we experience the wall as lighter in direct sunlight than where it is cast in shadow. For Kelly, the significance of this is that it is a case where there is a difference in the way we experience the wall in respect of color that is *not* a difference in which color we experience the wall as being. Color constancy demonstrates that there are differences in how experience presents things as being (in respect of color) that don't bear on which (color) concepts apply.

The broader significance of the phenomenon of color constancy, for Kelly, is that it shows that perceptual experience is context-dependent:

"The complete and accurate account of my perceptual experience of the color of an object must contain some reference to the lighting context in which that color is perceived" (2001, 607). No color concept, however fine-grained, can capture the ways in which experiences of one and the same color may differ; for these differences may not be differences in color. Even if it is true, then, that we have concepts of every color we can see, it still remains the case that color experiences can differ in color-relevant ways that don't correspond to differences in the application we can make of color concepts.

One response to this would be to observe that the context-dependent differences in color experience that Kelly has in mind all depend on the role of illumination. But the conceptualist can reply that these differences in experience are differences in conceptual content; the relevant concepts, however, are those of illumination, not color (Peacocke 2001).

A second response is more penetrating. Kelly writes: "If it is right, as all perceptual psychologists agree, that this change is not a change in color (hence the name "color constancy"), then no color concept, not even a demonstrative one, could completely capture the content of a color experience" (2001, 607). It may be true that all perceptual psychologists agree that there is color constancy (at least within a range of cases), but this doesn't do much to support Kelly's claim. The problem is that Kelly relies on a tendentious characterization of the phenomenon of color constancy. As argued in chapter 4 (see especially note 2, where I discuss Kelly's view), it is true that, in the imagined scenario, we can see that the wall is uniform in color. But this does not entail that we do not also see that the wall differs with respect to color across its surface. There is a clear and determinate sense in which the color is perceptibly nonuniform. For example, we would match the color of the wall *there* with one chip from a Munsell selection, and the color *over there* with a different chip. It is just misleading, then, to suggest that the difference in our experience of the color of the shaded part of the wall and the color of the directly illuminated part of the wall is not a difference in our experience of the wall's color. The enactive view explains this by suggesting that the actual color of the wall is precisely the way its appearance changes as color-critical conditions (e.g., illumination) change.

As discussed in chapter 5, perceptual content has a dual aspect. Factual content (how the experience presents things as being) can be distinguished from perspectival content (how things are presented as looking from a vantage point). The differences Kelly calls to our attention are differences in perspectival content, but precisely perspectival differences in our experience of *color*. These features are indeed context-dependent (after all, they are vantage-point-dependent, and vantage points are in large part what fixes a context, in the relevant sense). But there is no conflict between this context dependency and the fact that they are differences in apparent *color* (or apparent shape, etc.). What these considerations do not warrant, then, is the idea that these contextual factors need to be understood in nonconceptual terms.

6.9   Activity Trails

Adrian Cussins (2003), in considering matters closely related to those under discussion here, invites us to consider two different ways you can know how fast you are driving a motorcycle. One way of knowing how fast you are driving is to know, say, that you are driving 55 mph. In this case, as Cussins explains, your speed is given to you as a truth maker, that is, as something that makes it true that you are going 55 mph. The second way in which your speed can be given to you (in which you can know how fast you were going) is not as a truth maker, but, as it were, "as an element in a skilled interaction with the world, as a felt rotational pressure in my right hand as it held the throttle grip, a tension in my fingers and foot in contact with brake pedals or levers, a felt vibration of the road and a rush of wind, a visual rush of surfaces, a sense of how the immediate environment would *afford* certain motions and *resist* others; *embodied and environmental knowledge* of what it would take to make adjustments in these felt pressures and sensitivities" (Cussins 2003, 150).

Cussins uses this example to draw a distinction between what he calls *objectual* and *experiential* knowledge, and he suggests that the distinction runs deep. In objectual knowledge, the world is given to you as an independent domain of properties and states of affairs (a realm of reference), and thought about the world in this manner is governed by the norms of truth. In experiential knowledge, in contrast, the world is given to you not as an independent domain, but as affording possibilities for movement and action and experience, as, in Cussins's terms, a "domain of mediation." Your knowledge of your own speed, as you drive through the city, is a knowledge of an element in your interaction, and your knowledge of the city, as you drive along, is a knowledge of the city as made up of trails and paths and obstacles and roundabouts. Cussins thinks that objectual knowledge is conceptual—directed to truth and propositional representation—and that experiential knowledge is nonconceptual—directed to action and experience, not representation and truth.

The distinction between conceptual and nonconceptual content, for Cussins, then, is the distinction between knowledge for representation and knowledge for action. Experience presents the world not as a domain for thought, but as a domain for activity. The structure of activity is made up of *activity trails* that guide or lead one through environments of activity (as he explains).

Cussins's treatment of these issues is deep and original. He emphasizes that both forms of guidance—the guidance of truth, and that of activity—are basic and essential for our cognitive lives. Philosophical error, he thinks, comes in privileging one over the other. I am sympathetic to this approach. However, I don't think the distinction between objectional and experiential knowledge can be drawn so neatly, and I am unconvinced that we should think of experiential knowing as nonconceptual.

Thought and the pursuit of truth, after all, are also *activities*, structured by trails and possibilities of action. (Cussins implicitly recognizes this when he talks about trails in the laboratory.) And experience may be more complex as a result of its dual structure! Experience itself is directed to the world as affording opportunities for action, and also to the world as affording opportunities for thought.

One way to see this is to return to the motorcycle example. The relevant fact, I think, is that both ways of knowing how fast you were going are precisely that, ways of *knowing*, and they are both ways of knowing *how fast you're going*, that is, how things are. To recognize this, though, is to recognize that, at some level, these modes of awareness both structure the world as known the same way. And this squares with our commonsense ideas about the practical and the theoretical, too. So, for example, one can easily imagine a person being called on to testify as to how fast he was driving where the basis of his knowledge claim is experiential, not objectual. Music is an area where these two forms of knowledge seem to meet. You can understand musical facts and relationships even if you haven't studied music theory. The objectual knowledge is grounded in your skillful mastery of musical activity. And so is driving.

The significance of my objection to Cussins is this: It is a mistake to locate the important distinction in kinds of knowledge as a distinction between thought (the objectual, the world as a domain of reference) and perception (the experience, the world as mediating action). Rather, the crucial nearby distinction ought to be drawn *within* perceptual experience; it is the distinction between factual and perspectival dimensions of content I discussed in chapter 5. Experience presents us with how things are—for example, with deer grazing on the meadow—*and* it presents us with the world *as it appears from here.* If the argument of this book is right, it presents *how things are* because we understand the relation between how things are and the way how things appear changes as we move. This understanding is sensorimotor, but it is, crucially, a form of understanding.

Cussins's distinction nicely marks the difference between practical endeavors, on the one hand (such as swimming, games playing, etc.), and theoretical inquiry, on the other. Experience itself, however, cannot be easily placed in one or the other of these categories. Indeed, it encompasses both. Experience, I have argued, is *thoughtful activity.*

6.10 Understanding in the Natural World

In this final section, I speculate about the basis of conceptual skill. One of the arguments for nonconceptual content—one that I've ignored until now—is empiricist in its basic form: Concepts stand to each other in asymmetrical relations. Some concepts are such that to understand them we must understand simpler concepts out of which they are, as it were, composed. So, for example, to understand the geometrical concept *square,* you must understand the concepts *line,* say, and *angle.* You don't need to know what a square is, however, to grasp what a line is. It would seem to follow then that there are some concepts whose application is so basic that they do not depend on the thinker's possession of any other concepts. They are applied, when they are applied by someone who grasps them, not in circumstances in which a range of constitutive concepts apply, but rather, simply, when they apply. The basis of such concepts must be nonconceptual.

Peacocke, who has explored this line of thought (in Peacocke 1992), suggests that perceptual concepts (*observational* concepts) may be primitive and rest on a nonconceptual basis in just this way. To understand the concept *red*, say, one must know that it is correctly applied in the face (as it were) of the right kind of experiences (experiences with the right kind of qualitative character), and for the reason that one has experiences of this sort. But there is no requirement that one must have concepts of the qualitative character of the experiences in question. With these experiences one has, as it were, reached bedrock, and there is no further need for understanding. Part of what motivates this claim, on Peacocke's part, is the recognition that there are no candidate concepts in the offing that we can use to conceptualize the experience on the basis of which we experience something as red. What sort of concept might we make use of to conceptualize the experience itself? The standard move, historically, is to characterize the experience as one of, say, something's *looking red*. But the problem here is clear. We haven't succeeded in explaining what our grasp of *red* consists in if we suppose that it consists in our prior grasp of *looks red*. For we don't have an independent or prior grasp of *looks red*, as distinct from *red*.

Peacocke makes similar claims for the primitiveness of nonperceptual concepts as well, for example, logical concepts of simple inferences. So, for example, one who understands modus ponens is disposed to infer q from if p then q and p precisely on the basis of the primitive grasp of modus ponens, not on the basis of anything more primitive.

We are now in a position to criticize Peacocke's account of perceptual concepts. First, we have already (in chapter 4) rejected the idea that there are simple qualia whose presence governs the application of color concepts. Second, and more immediately related to the themes of this chapter, the ground of perceptual or observational concepts is not so much nonconceptual as it is sensorimotor. To experience something as cubical, on an observational basis, is to experience it as something disposed to vary in a special way under actual and possible movements. These principles or laws of sensorimotor contingency are not dependent on my prior possession of the concept of *cube* but rather partially constitute it.

Consider, once again, the familiar standoff on the matter of sense data. The sense-datum theorist denies that we really see the whole cube, insisting that we *go beyond* what is given in our experience when we characterize it as an experience *as of* a cube. For the cube, in its three-dimensionality, isn't *given*. The direct realist replies that the experience is indeed given to us precisely in terms of cube presence. To extract cube presence from the experience does not leave you with experience of raw sense data. It leaves you with nothing remotely resembling experience as of anything at all. For it is the concept *cube* that gives *content* to the experience.

We have seen that the direct realist cannot be entirely right. There *is* a sense in which it is not possible to see the whole cube; we see only its facing side. But crucially—and this is where the direct realist pulls ahead again—the sense of the presence of the whole cube is *sensory*. It is *as if* we see it all (even though, of course, it is impossible to see it all). The understanding that gives us the three-dimensional presence of the cube is a kind of *sensorimotor* understanding. In this way, our possession of sensorimotor knowledge is the basis of our possession of the observational concept *cube*.

In chapter 2 I observed that our sense of the occluded portion of a tomato contrasts with our sense of the presence of the room next door (in making this observation, I was building on O'Regan and Noë 2001a,b). Our relation to the tomato is mediated by sensorimotor relations (e.g., blinking and head turning makes a difference), whereas our relation to the room next door is mediated merely by thought (blinking and head turning make no difference). The *sensory* quality of the presence of the side of the tomato is thus explained in contradistinction to the merely thought presence of the room next door.

Of course it is clear that the line here is not sharp. After all, as I mentioned in chapter 2, sensorimotor relations mediate my relation to the room next door as well. I could get up and move my body and turn my head and thus bring it into view. The presence of a thing *as thought* and the presence of a thing *as experienced* are, in this sense, different not in kind, but only in degree.

This suggests the stronger possibility that our relation to the world, through thought, and our relation to it through experience, differ not in kind, but in degree. Poincaré perhaps had this sort of consideration in mind when he argued that the basis of our grasp on *absolute space* is our grasp of our bodily, egocentric spaces. Empiricists, like Hume, Carnap, and the Vienna Circle, were right that experience of the world is the ground of thought about the world. If the suggestion we are entertaining is right, though, they misunderstood the significance of this fact. What is primitive are not sensory qualities (sensations, ideas, whatever). What is primitive is sensorimotor understanding. But sensorimotor understanding is just that, a kind of understanding. The root of our ability to think about the world is our ability to experience it; but experience is a mode of skillful encounter.

7 Brain in Mind: A Conclusion

We are told that vision depends on the eye, which is connected to the brain. I shall suggest that natural vision depends on the eyes in the head on a body supported by the ground, the brain being only the central organ of a complete visual system.
—James J. Gibson

7.1 Explanatory Gaps

Most cognitive scientists hold that for every experience there is a neural structure or substrate whose activation is sufficient for the experience. On this way of thinking, experiences are internal biological processes, comparable to digestion or respiration; they happen inside us. Philosophers sometimes put the basic idea like this: Neural duplicates are necessarily experiential duplicates, for experience *supervenes* on states of the brain.

In this final chapter I want to question this doctrinal consensus. Even to do this will strike some readers as silly and a waste of time. Isn't it just plain obvious that experience is what happens as a result of the way the world affects us? Discussing the enactive approach to consciousness, for example, Christof Koch writes: "If there is one thing that scientists are reasonably sure of, it is that brain activity is both necessary and sufficient for biological sentience . . . action is not necessary for consciousness . . . behavior is not strictly necessary for qualia to occur" (2004, sec. 1.2). In a similar vein, John Searle takes the solution to the mind-body problem to be simple and "consistent with everything we know about biology and about how the world works. It is this: Consciousness and other sorts of mental phenomena are caused by neurobiological processes in the brain, and they are realized in the structure of the brain. In a word, the conscious mind is caused by brain processes and is itself a higher level feature of the brain" (2000, 566).

The very confidence with which these assertions are made is, I suspect, a giveaway that the "consciousness is in the head" doctrine is not so much a working hypothesis as it is an assumed starting point. But this is to get ahead of ourselves. Whether or not neural activity is alone sufficient for an experience is, or at least ought to be regarded as, an empirical question. On what empirical basis, let us then ask, is the issue taken to have been settled?

Our question is not unmotivated. As of now, there is no account, even in roughest outline, of how the brain produces consciousness. This is widely admitted, even by leading proponents of the "consciousness is in the head" point of view, such as neurobiologists Frances Crick and Christof Koch. They write: "No one has produced any plausible explanation as to how the experience of the redness of red could arise from the action of the brain" (Crick and Koch 2003, 119). In light of this "explanatory gap," talk of neural substrates of experience can seem empty. Beyond brute correlation, we lack any intelligible connection between neural substrate and experience, and so we lack, it seems, sufficient reason to believe, of any given neural structure, that it is or could be the substrate of an experience.[1]

In this final chapter I explore the implications of the enactive approach to perception and consciousness for our understanding of the neural basis of experience.[2] In particular, I argue that many of the reasons given for adopting "internalism" about perceptual experience—the "consciousness is in the head" model—are weak and unpersuasive. I argue that the strongest motivation for the internalist "fallback position" may be reliance on bad phenomenology; there is no a priori obstacle to the possibility that experience might depend constitutively on physical substrates that are not inside the head (e.g., on dynamic patterns of interaction among neural processes, the body, and the environment). Finally, I argue that there may in fact be good reasons to entertain the possibility that this is sometimes the case: Neural activity may not be sufficient to account for the character of *some* experiences (or for some aspects of many experiences).

7.2   Are Experiences in the Head? A First Pass

It is sometimes suggested that the fact that neuroscientists can produce sensations by direct stimulation of the brain shows that consciousness is a matter of what is going on in the head alone (e.g., by Koch 2004, sec. 1.2). But there are two reasons to doubt this.

First, we need to be careful not to rely too heavily on science fiction. We are now able to produce very simple visual sensations such as the illusion of the presence of flashes of light ("phosphenes") by means of direct neural stimulation (as shown by Penfield; see Penfield and Jasper 1954). At the present time, however, we are not able directly to generate more complicated experiences. The first point to make, then, is that from the fact that it is possible to produce *some* experiences, it does not follow that it is possible to produce *all* experiences. To assume, without further discussion, that we will someday be able to produce all perceptual experiences by direct neural stimulation, or that it is in principle possible to do so, is to assume too much. Indeed, it is to come close to assuming internalism about experience.

Second, even if we suppose that some not-yet-invented technology will one day allow us to produce by direct neural intervention *any* perceptual experience, that would not in itself show that neural states were sufficient for experience. Consider a comparison: The states of a car's engine are necessary conditions of its driving activity; moreover, in certain conditions one can change the car's driving behavior by directly modulating the states of its engine. But it is absurd to think that the states of the engine are alone sufficient for driving! The engine needs to be properly embodied in the vehicle, and the car itself must be situated in an appropriate environment. A car suspended from a hook, or up to its windows in mud, won't drive, no matter what the state of the engine. (See figure 7.1.)

In general, just as the fact that one can manipulate the car's behavior by manipulating its engine is not enough to show that the engine is alone sufficient for the car's behavior, so the fact that one can manipulate experience by manipulating the brain is not enough to show that the brain is sufficient for experience. At most it would show that experience could be produced by means of interaction between a probing scientist and a healthy animal. We haven't yet imagined a case in which experience emerges from the causal effects of neural activity alone.

Given that, as a matter of fact, we spend our lives in tight coupling with the environment (and other people), one can reasonably wonder why we find it so plausible that there could be a consciousness like ours independent of active exchange with the world? Why are we so certain consciousness depends only on what is going on inside us?

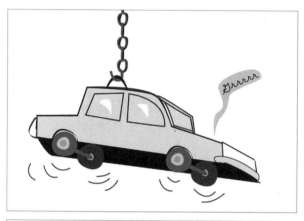

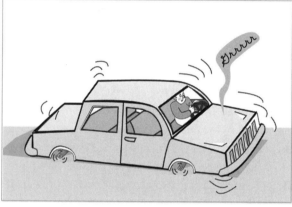

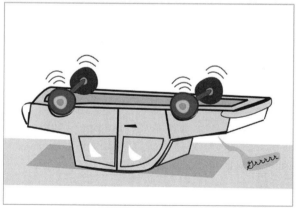

Figure 7.1
A car's ability to drive 70 mph depends on the manner of its situation in the environment.

Defenders of the "consciousness is in the head" thesis may at this stage refer to dreaming (as Koch 2004, sec. 1.2 does; Searle, personal communication). The fact that we dream, they may say, shows that experience depends only on what is going on in the head. For when we dream, they add, we are not engaged in dynamic patterns of interaction with the world.

This is a classic maneover in the repertoire of the internalist. It packs prestige as a rhetorical move and is sometimes taken to be an argument stopper. But what does it really demonstrate?

Let us take it as settled that when we dream there is no dynamic exchange with the environment (although this might turn out not to be true), and let us accept that, therefore, neural states alone *are* sufficient for dreaming (although this does not follow—e.g., the affective content of dream states *may* depend on endocrine gland activity, as waking emotional states do; see Damasio 1994, 15). Given these assumptions, what the fact of dreaming shows is *not* that neural activity alone is sufficient for perceptual experience, but only that it is sufficient for *dreaming* experience.

At this point the internalist will snort with pleasure and take it that the battle is won, because, he or she will assert, dream experiences and normal perceptual experiences are, or at least sometimes can be, qualitatively identical. Historical authority and tradition provide heft to this phenomenological claim. Ever since Descartes it has been widely assumed that there is no way, from within perceptual consciousness, to determine whether or not one is dreaming. There are no differences, it is thought, between dreaming and non-dreaming consciousness.

I do not claim to be able to offer a satisfactory reply to Descartes' dream-based argument for external world skepticism. But that's not necessary. Crucially, Descartes' argument does not turn on there being qualitative identity between dreaming states and nondreaming states; rather it turns on the fact that, in the first person, there is no way to be sure that one is not the victim of a dreamlike hallucination. Importantly, from the fact that it is impossible to tell for sure whether one is dreaming or seeing, it doesn't follow that there is no experiential difference between dreaming and seeing (a point made by Austin [1962, 48–49]; and also more recently by Putnam [1999, 153]). Just as the fact that one may not be able to tell two twins apart does not mean there aren't visible differences in their appearances, so the fact that a dreamer may think he or she is waking is not evidence that there are no differences between waking and dreaming experience.

Setting aside the skeptical context, there *are* reasons to believe that differences exist between dream visual experiences and non-dream visual experiences. The biggest difference, phenomenologically speaking, has to do with detail and stability. Dream sequences tend to be poor in detail, and what detail there is tends to vary unstably across scenes.[3] Perhaps this is explained by the fact that, as a neuroscientific matter, the brain is not very good at storing detailed representations of scenes. In normal perception, there is no need to store detail, since the world is available to serve as a repository of information about itself. This suggests a hypothesis: Dream states are unstable and poor in detail precisely because dream states, unlike normal, non-dream perceptual states, *are* produced by neural activity alone. Actual perceptual consciousness is anchored by the fact that we interact with, refer to, and have access to the environment. The stability of the environment is what gives our experiences their familiar stability. The stability of normal experience is explained by the involvement of the world in our experience.

These speculations aside, the appeal to dreaming doesn't *settle* anything in favor of the internalist. It does, however, give us further reason to suspect that the "consciousness is in the head" doctrine has Cartesian fingerprints all over it. Again, we can wonder whether internalism is less a working hypothesis than a philosophical preconception. Whatever we say about this, the battle is *not* over.

At this stage the defender of what I am increasingly inclined to think of as the *dogma* of internalism may feel inclined to warn that the alternative to the idea that neural states are the sufficient basis for experience is dualism or plain mystery. But playing the dualism card is unwarranted. Consider our example of the car again. From the fact that the states of the car's engine are not sufficient for the driving behavior of the car, it does not follow that the car's driving depends on unnatural processes in an immaterial medium! Nor would the recognition that neural activity is not sufficient for consciousness require retreat to an unscientific spiritualism. The brain is one element in a complex network involving the brain, the body, and the environment (just as the car's engine is one element in a system made up of engine, driver, vehicle, and environmental setting).

Descartes wrote that the mind is not lodged in the body the way a pilot is lodged in his ship (Descartes [1641] 1988a); the connection is tighter than that. Descartes was unable to come up with a satisfying account of what the connection is. Are contemporary neuroscientists working on consciousness faring any better? It's worth asking whether they aren't making just the mistake that Descartes warned against: They treat the mind as standing to the body as a pilot does to his ship and they deceive themselves into thinking they've eliminated mystery because they use the word "mind" to refer to the brain. The brain, thought of in this way, is less material mind than spiritualized matter; instead of eliminating the mystery from the mental, they've simply concocted a mysterious account of the physical.

In the next sections, I try to show how a plausible externalism about experience might go. My argument turns on the implications of the enactive way of understanding the character of perceptual experience that I have been developing in this book.

7.3   Virtual Content

In chapters 2 and 4 I argued that perceptual content is thoroughly virtual. The upshot of this claim, I argued (see chapter 4), is that it is a mistake to factor experience into an occurrent and a merely potential or dispositional aspect. I now want to propose that the virtual character of perceptual content and quality is the basis for an argument that at least sometimes "the environment can drive and so partially constitute" our perceptual experience (Clark and Chalmers 1998).

Let us revisit the idea that perceptual experience is virtual.

The content of a perceptual experience is not given all at once the way the content of a picture is given in the picture all at once, as discussed in chapter 2. I have a sense of the visual presence of the detailed scene before me, even though it is not the case that I see all that detail (or that I think that I can see it all). As a matter of phenomenology, the detail is present not *as represented*, but *as accessible*. Experience has content as a potentiality. In this sense, the detail is present perceptually in my experience *virtually*. Thanks to my possession of sensorimotor and cognitive skills, I have access to nearby detail.

If the content of experience is virtual, in this way, then there is *a sense* in which the content of experience is not in the head. Nor is it in the world. Experience isn't something that happens in us. It is something we do; it is a temporally extended process of skillful probing. The world makes itself available to our reach. The experience comprises mind and world. Experience has content only thanks to the established dynamics of interaction between perceiver and world.

But this is much too quick as an argument against the "consciousness-is-in-the-head" dogma. The very metaphor of "virtual" content invites the objection that all that is present in your computer, *really*, is what is already downloaded. Information on the network is accessible, but it isn't really present. The illusion of presence depends only on the current state of your local machine. Similar claims can be made about perception. Granted that perceptual experience depends on expectations of the sensory effects of movement. This just shows that these expectations need to be accounted for in the current state of your brain. Anyone with a brain identical to yours would have the sense of presence of the same variety of features, even if their environment were radically different than yours!

This is a compelling line of objection. Here is how I think we should respond to it. First, as developed in chapter 4, phenomenologically speaking, virtual presence is a kind of presence, not a kind of non-presence or illusory presence. My sense of the perceptual presence of items at the periphery of my visual field, or of partially occluded items, is not a sense that I actually see these features, but that I have access to them, due to the fact that my relation to them is mediated by patterns of sensorimotor contingency.

Second, as argued in chapter 4, experiential presence is virtual *all the way in*. Experience is fractal and dense. Wherever you look in your visual field, at whatever scale you select, you are always given a whole field that contains elements that are focal, and elements that are peripheral, elements that are surveyable, and elements that are hidden. When you peel away the layers of potentiality and merely virtual presence, you are not left with pure phenomenal content, that which, as it were, is present to your mind now. You are always presented with qualities that in turn have qualities and that are presented against a structured background.

This is an important disanalogy with the computer case. Consider the tomato again. You see the facing side. You can't see the far side, but you have a perceptual sense of its presence thanks to your practical grasp of sensorimotor patterns mediating your relation to it. The rear side is present virtually, but the facing side is simply present. Notice, however, that you do not, as a matter of fact, have the *whole* of the facing side of the tomato in consciousness all at once. The facing side has extent and shape and color, and you can't embrace all this detail in consciousness all at once, any more than you can embrace the whole detailed scene. This is clear to careful consideration. Take a tomato out. Look at it. Yes, you have a sense that the facing side of the tomato is all there, all at once. But if you are careful you will admit that you don't actually experience every part even of its visible surface all at once. Your eyes scan the surface, and you direct your attention to this or that. Further evidence is provided by change blindness. As discussed in chapters 2 and 4, the very color of the object you are staring at can change right before your eyes without your noticing it, so long as you are not attending to the color itself!

What this shows, as stated, is that you cannot factor experience into an occurrent and a merely potential part. Pick any candidate for the occurrent factor. Now consider it. It too is structured; it too has hidden facets or aspects. It is present only in potiential.

Qualities are available in experience as possibilities, as potentialities, but not as completed givens. Experience is a dynamic process of navigating the pathways of these possibilities. Experience depends on the skills needed to make one's way.

The upshot of this is that there is no basis, in phenomenology at least, for thinking that what is given now, to me, as present in my consciousness, is ever enough to account exhaustively for the character of my current conscious experience. My phenomenal experience expands my immediate horizons and takes me beyond myself to the world. This sounds paradoxical, but it is not. Presence in absence, as we considered in chapter 2, is a pervasive feature of our perceptual lives. Phenomenology (at least) is compatible with externalism about perceptual experience.

7.4 Are Experiences in the Head?

"Does experience supervene on internal states of the brain?" The correct answer to this ought to be "maybe." I have argued that what we experience outstrips what is represented in consciousness. This *does not* entail that what we experience outstrips what is represented in our brains. However, it does remove the major theoretical obstacle to entertaining the possibility that experience might supervene not on the brain, but rather on brain-animal-world systems. *It is an empirical question whether our brains can do the work needed to enable us to enact our virtual worlds.* For example, it is an empirical question whether the brain can store and organize the information about the world needed to supply the content of experience. It is a mistake—a prejudice really—to think these questions have already been settled.

"Wouldn't my neural duplicate have the same experiences as I do?" Perhaps, but your neural duplicate would almost certainly be embedded in and interacting with a duplicate of your environment. What else could explain the neural identity? (This point has been discussed by Hurley [1998]; see also Hurley and Noë 2003a.) But wouldn't my neural duplicate have the same experiences as me *whatever differences there might be between its environment and mine?* This is the force of the claim that experience supervenes on the brain.

Again, this is an empirical question. If, as I have suggested, experience frequently makes use of temporally extended, dynamic access to the world, then it comes down to the question of whether brains can suffice without actual reference to the world itself. There is some reason to think that they cannot. This is one way to interpret the change blindness findings. Without reliable access to the detail around us, we lose track of detail. We don't have access to a world model in the head.

We can actually make a stronger point: If experience is temporally extended in the way I have suggested, then a neural duplicate of me now, at a moment in time, won't, by dint of being my duplicate now, have *any* experience at all (as Mark Rowlands has called to my attention in correspondence). If the duplicate does have experience, it will be owing to its dynamic, temporally extended interaction with the environment. But then again we must note that there is little reason to think that its experience would or could be like mine unless its environment were also like mine.

A reasonable bet, at this point, is that *some* experience, or some features of some experiences, are, as it were, exclusively neural in their causal basis, but that full-blown, mature human experience is not. This is supported by such facts as that, until now, neuroscientists have been able to produce only relatively primitive experiences by direct stimulation of the cortex (Koch 2004). More important, it is just not clear, given the virtual character of perceptual content, why an internal representation would be any better than access to the world itself. This harkens back to Wittgenstein's idea that anything a picture in the head could do could be done by a picture held in the hand. We go a step further: Why do we need a picture at all? The world is right there, after all. We are *in the world*. We have the skills needed to enact our perceptual experience.[4]

The computer comparison may help again: My desktop may have enough memory to allow me to download the entire online version of *The New York Times* at one go. No need to make use of dynamic, networked access. But maybe I don't know how to do that, or maybe my desktop isn't big enough to allow such a big download, or maybe doing that would interfere with my computer's performance in other ways. Or perhaps, although I *could* do that, I choose not to because doing so would mean I would miss out on the constant updates that are provided online.

It always seemed that there were obstacles to thinking that consciousness (in contrast with cognition) could extend beyond the limits of the skull. "Gosh darn it, experience just feels like it's in the head." But this is bad phenomenology, I have argued, and it is probably bad science. As we have seen, detail may be present in consciousness only virtually. We thus open up the possibility of an account of, for example, the perceptual experience of detail that is consistent with its not being the case that that detail is represented at once in the head. Although of course it *could* be. The upshot is not that experience is without the head, but that it might be. The world is safe for an externalism that allows that we enact perceptual content by the exercise of sensorimotor skills over time.

7.5   Searle's Objection

The gist of the discussion so far, then, is that experience might not be in the head. Whether it is depends on whether, as a matter of fact, the causal basis of experience depends on ongoing, causal interaction among brain, body, and environment. I have urged that there is nothing in our phenomenology that should lead us to accept an internalist position on this.

Searle (2004) has argued that the controversy between internalism and externalism frequently turns on a failure to distinguish different ways of describing experiences. One can describe experiences in an idiom that appeals to public places, properties, actions, and so forth, as, for example, when one reflects on the experience of a pleasurable dinner with friends in a country inn. But the very same experience can be redescribed in a way that brackets reference to the inn and the food and the company and instead focuses only on the experienced qualities and internal events produced inside one while enjoying the food and the wine and the conversation. To think that these internal goings-on are constituted by anything external, Searle suggests, would be like supposing that digestion is external because as a process it requires the presence of food. We can describe digestion in a food-involving way, or we can describe it as an internal process that unfolds once the food is ingested, that is, made internal. On Searle's view, experiences are internal in just the way that digestion is (and they can be thought of as world-involving in the same way). Searle is also quick to add that he doesn't wish his advocacy of an idea of experience as internal to get confused with anything like the old sense-datum theory. In particular, he is not committed to the idea that the internal states can themselves be described in a sense-datum language. It happens to be the case that the only way we have to characterize our internal experiences, even to ourselves, is by means of a public, shared language.

Searle's claims are compatible with its being the case that experiences are external in my sense, that is, that they depend on causal interactions between the animal and its environment. Searle's observations do not address what is, in the present context, the basic question: What *is* the causal substrate of the experience of the wine's flavor? Perhaps this substrate is only neural, but perhaps it is not. For example, perhaps the only way—or the only biologically possible way—to produce just the flavor sensations one enjoys when one sips a wine is by rolling a liquid across one's tongue. In that case, the liquid, the tongue, and the rolling action would be part of the physical substrate for the experience's occurrence.

A comparison may help: Sometimes we calculate "in our heads," but sometimes we calculate with a pencil and paper. Indeed, for a great many calculations that we can perform, the pencil and paper are necessary. If the pencil and paper are necessary for the calculation, why not view them as part of the necessary substrate for the calculating activity? This point was entertained by Wittgenstein (1958) and has recently been elaborated by Clark and Chalmers (1998), who defend what they call "active externalism." Some cognitive states—for example, states of thinking, calculating, navigating—may be partially external because, at least sometimes, these states depend on the use of symbols and artifacts that are outside the body. Maps, signs, and writing implements may sometimes be as inextricably bound up with the workings of cognition as neural structures or internally realized symbols (if there are any). According to active externalism, the environment can drive and so partially constitute cognitive processes. Where does the mind stop and the rest of the world begin? If active externalism is right, then the boundary cannot be drawn at the skull. The mind reaches—or at least *can* reach, *sometimes*—beyond the limits of the body out into the world.

Active externalism relies on a distinction drawn by Dennett (1991; see also Hurley 1998, chap. 1) between the content of a state and that content's *vehicle*. In general, Dennett argues, it is a mistake to think you can read off properties of vehicles of content (e.g., neural structures and systems, or sentences for that matter) from the contents of the resulting states. The experience of a cube needn't be carried by a cubical neural structure of vehicle. One way to frame the claim of active externalism is as a form of externalism about the vehicles or carriers of content (Hurley 1998): In some cases, Clark and Chalmers argue, the vehicles of content cross boundaries, looping out of the head into the world.

What I have been defending in this chapter is externalism about the vehicles of content of experience.[5] I have been arguing that, for at least some experiences, the physical substrate of the experience *may* cross boundaries, implicating neural, bodily, and environmental features. Just as Clark and Chalmers have argued that there is no theoretical obstacle to thinking that the vehicles of some *cognitive* processes may cross the boundary of the skull, so I am arguing that the vehicles of some *experience* too may extend out into the world (but not that it must do so). Nothing in what Searle says—about the fact that it is possible to reflect on one's experiences in a way that brackets them off from their distal causes—weighs against this. Crucially, on the externalism I am defending here, a number of home truths of internalism are left undisturbed. For example, the *enactive externalism* I defend here is compatible with its being the case that the only way the world produces changes in animal consciousness is by producing changes in the brain; that appropriate changes in the brain will produce changes in consciousness, even if the environment is unchanged. Indeed, the externalism I defend here is compatible with its being the case that neural duplicates will be duplicates with respect to consciousness. Crucially, it hasn't yet been shown that this last claim is true; if it were true, it's worth noting, that wouldn't entail that neural states *were* sufficient for experience, for we haven't yet given content to the supposition that you could have neural duplicates in the absence of duplication of patterns of interaction with the environment.

Searle has stressed (in conversation and in his writings) that if you want to learn more about why a creature embedded in such and such an environment has precisely the experiences it has, it makes sense to look inward, to the neural plumbing that makes the experience possible. I agree with this. But it also makes sense to look outward, too, to the way that plumbing is hooked up to the world. It may be that we can only get the kind of explanations we seek when we take this wider perspective.

Searle makes another point in this arena that is important and that I want to endorse. He writes:

Most of the discussions that I have seen of the NCC [neural correlates of consciousness] are confused because the researchers are looking for an NCC for a particular element of the conscious field, such as, for example, the experience of the color red. But that experience occurs in a subject who is already conscious. So the NCC could not possibly give us sufficient conditions for consciousness because the subject has to be already conscious in order that the NCC in question can cause a particular perceptual experience. The basic insight is this: We should not think of perception as creating consciousness, but as modifying the preexisting conscious field. That is why most of the research that I have seen does not give an NCC but what we might call us a NCPP—a neural correlate of a particular perception, *given that the subject is already conscious.* (Searle 2004, 80–81)

Searle argues here that the neural substrate of a given particular perceptual experience will never be nomically sufficient for the occurrence of that experience, for it gives rise to the experience only given the background of the subject's consciousness. That's exactly right. In my opinion, however, Searle stops short at recognizing the most significant consequence of this: Consciousness is a phenomenon that occurs only against the background of the active life of the animal. There is no good reason for assuming that the only relevant background is the activity of the brain.

7.6   Supervenience and Time

Seeing, on the enactive view, is like painting (a point articulated in chapter 5). When a painter works from life, he or she makes continuous and ongoing reference to the world. The painter looks to the world, then back to the canvas, then back to the world, then back to the canvas. Eye, hand, canvas, paint, world are brought into play in the process of constructing the picture. Seeing, like painting, involves the temporally extended process of reaching out and probing the scene. The causally sufficient substrate of the production of the picture is surely not the internal states of the painter, but rather the dynamic pattern of engagement among the painter, the scene, and the canvas. Why not say the same thing about seeing? Seeing, on this approach, would depend on brain, body, and world.

The internalist may respond that I have succeeded only in showing that perceptual experience is a temporally extended process, as such it may depend on a temporally extended series of brain states. I haven't shown, so the internalist will insist, that the causal substrate of experience is without the head, that experience depends causally on physical processes involving the extra-neural world.[6] If experience is temporally extended, then experience must supervene on a temporal series of brain states. Any possible world in which that temporal series of brain states were to occur would be a world in which just that experience was had.

But is this so? It may be that the only nomically possible world in which such a temporal series of brain states could occur would be one in which the animal were dynamically interacting with the very same kind of environment! To imagine the duplication of brain states is thus tacitly to appeal to the more extended setting in which those brain states are placed. Experience doesn't supervene on neural states alone, then, but only on neural states plus environmental conditions.

A defender of internalism will not accept this. It is just not the case that the only possible worlds in which dynamic patterns of neural activity would be duplicated would also be worlds in which local environments were duplicated. One can imagine, so the objector continues, a "virtual reality" world in which perceivers received the same sensory input and sensorimotor feedback as they would in a normal environment despite sitting in a darkened room with goggles on.[7] This would be a world in which the local environment was radically different but the internal states of the organism were the same. If we admit that experience would be the same in this imagined scenario, then we are admitting that what determines experience is what is going on in the head, not what is going on in the world. Indeed, in a case such as this, the objector continues, we can explain why experience is the same: The two different environments both produce the same internal effects on the brain; the brain generates the same experiences.

But this is much too fast. The enactive externalist need hardly be committed to the impossibility of virtual reality (although it is worth noticing that virtual reality systems, real ones, do make use of actual, embodied movement, so there is no elimination of the non-brain body). Nor need the enactive externalist be committed to the impossiblity of radical hallucination or misperception. All the externalist is committed to is the possibility that neural states alone are not sufficient for the experience; indeed, that there is reason to think that this possibility might be actual, at least for some aspects of experience. The virtual world counterexample doesn't effectively challenge this commitment.

To see why, consider that in the virtual world scenario we do not consider neural states giving rise to experience in isolation. Rather, we consider neural systems embedded in and interacting with a network of inputs (and thus eliciting outputs) carefully engineered by the designers of the system. It is this dynamic causal interaction that allows for experience with a given content. There's no way to treat this as a case illustrating the sufficiency of neural states alone for experience.

In reply, the internalist is likely to assert that all that internalism requires is that neural duplicates in *different* environments have the same experiential states. That's enough to show that what determines or explains the sameness of the experience cannot be the sameness of the environment but must be the sameness of neural states.

The enactive externalist has a few different points to make in reply to this. First, the virtual world and the actual world are, in the example we are considering, similar. This is in part because the virtual world is designed to resemble the actual world. In particular, the virtual world is such that one's conceptual and sensorimotor skills are easily drawn into play; one's readiness to apply them extends to the virtual scenario. For this reason, then, the virtual reality scenario does not provide an example of sameness of experience despite difference in (or indeed the absence of) the environment. The virtual world is precisely a virtual *world*. That is, it is an environment set up to resemble the nonvirtual world.

Second, it is impossible to know, a priori, or on any other basis, whether neural duplicates in different environments (virtual or otherwise) could have qualitatively identical experiential states. In the non–"virtual reality" case, it's impossible to know how things would be for subjects in a world in which neural states were insulated from dynamic interaction with the environment in the way that is being imagined. In our world, as noted previously, it is reasonable to say that neural duplicates would be experiential duplicates, but that's in part because, in our world, neural duplicates would find themselves in duplicate environments (at least in the relevant respects).

In the virtual reality case, it is likewise impossible to know whether you would get sameness of experience. Certainly that isn't the case with our current virtual reality systems. Here we run up against the sort of puzzle that entertained Borges, who pondered maps built to the same scale as the worlds they modeled. Such maps would be useless *as* maps. The relevant point here is that one can reasonably wonder whether one could ever produce a true virtual reality; to do so would require the reduplication of the degrees of freedom of movement, thought, and expectation of our actual reality, and that may be unfeasible. In any case, for the reasons considered earlier, it is not clear whether the possibility of virtual reality actually undercuts the externalist point. For, in the relevant respects, a virtual world would be just that, a world, a repository of information external to the living being, whose presence and availability is a condition on the possibility of experience with mature content.

If it is true that neural duplicates would have the same experiences *regardless* of their environmental embedding, then it would seem that the neural sufficiency thesis was true in some significant degree.[8] But what reasons have been given for thinking that it is true? None! The assertion of the supposed possibility of experiential duplicates is just a way of reasserting the "consciousness is in the head" dogma. And that brings us back to the beginning. Why should we accept this dogma?

7.7 Toward an Enactive Neuroscience of Perception

The enactive approach operates at two distinct levels. On the one hand, the approach, as I have developed it throughout this book, is meant to offer an explanation of why perceptual experience is the way it is. As we have seen, similarities and differences among sensory modalities, and differences in perceptual content within a modality, are explained in terms of the different kinds of sensorimotor skills perceivers draw on in their exploratory activity. (These ideas are a central theme of O'Regan and Noë 2001a,b, and Hurley and Noë 2003a,b; Noë and Hurley 2003) The theory aims, in this sense, to offer an *explanation* of perceptual consciousness, to be explanatorily adequate.

On the other hand, the theory is meant to be phenomenologically apt. It seeks to do justice to our phenomenology. For example, it proposes to explain perceptual phenomena—such as the visual experience of shape, the experience of detail, color experience—in a manner that is intuitively plausible and satisfying. Consider, for example, what the approach says about TVSS. TVSS is a quasi-visual modality because TVSS and vision share a common sensorimotor structure (O'Regan and Noë 2001a; Noë 2002a; Hurley and Noë 2003a,b).

The enactive approach provides explanation—of, for example, the qualitative similarity of TVSS and vision—where neural accounts alone are explanatorily afloat. In this way, the enactive approach tries to bridge the explanatory gap by expanding our conception of the substrate in terms of which we hope to explain consciousness (Hurley and Noë 2003a). Instead of framing explanation in neural terms, the view directs us to examine the way neural systems subserve the activity of the embodied and embedded animal. As in the Gibson passage given as the epigraph to this chapter, the enactive approach views neural activity as one important and indeed central element in a system involving the brain, the body, and the world (Gibson 1979, 1).

Hurley and I have argued (Hurley and Noë 2003a,b; Noë and Hurley 2003), for example, that neural rewiring leads to experiential plasticity (changes in the character of experience) only when the rewiring plays a role in a process of sensorimotor reintegration. Crucially, the qualitative character of experience may not be determined by the intrinsic properties of neural activity set up by stimulation in one region or another, but rather by the way that neural activity is integrated into dynamic patterns of sensorimotor looping (Hurley and Noë 2003a,b,c). The enactive approach thus allows us to explain why neural activity in occipital lobe (in visual cortex) can subserve tactile experience in blind readers of Braille (as shown by Pascual-Leone and Hamilton [2001]; e.g., Sadato et al. 1996, 1998; Buchel 1998; Buchel et al. 1998) and also why TMS (transcranial magnetic stimulation) applied to occipital lobe in blind readers can produce *tactile* illusions (Cohen et al. 1997). The approach also explains why somatosensory activity can subserve quasi-visual experience in TVSS. Indeed, Hurley and I (Hurley and Noë 2003a) predict that TMS to somatosensory cortex in TVSS ought to generate quasi-visual spatial distortions. The sort of enactive, dynamic sensorimotor approach we favor provides a nice framework within which to understand the work of Mriganka Sur and colleagues on auditory rewiring in ferrets (Roe et al. 1990, 1992; Pallas and Sur 1993; Sur, Angelucci, and Sharma 1999; Sharma, Angelucci, and Sur, 2000; Merzenich 2000). Appropriately embedded in a "visual" sensorimotor dynamic, neural activity in "auditory" cortex in young ferrets takes on "visual" functions.[9]

These are all instances of full-blooded perceptual plasticity. But neural rewiring does not always lead to plasticity in this way. For example, when neurons in "face cortex" in amputees invade neighboring cortical regions normally dedicated to the hand, many subjects report the feeling of being touched in the (phantom) hand when the face is touched. Why don't we get plasticity here as well? Why doesn't "hand cortex" modulate its qualitative effects, taking on "touch to face" properties, in the way that, say, visual cortex can take on tactile function, or somatosensory cortex can take on visual function? Hurley and I offer the following explanation: The patterns of neural activity in hand cortex that results from rewiring are not integrated in a dynamic pattern of sensorimotor dependence set up by the animal's activity.[10] In general, what determines phenomenology is not neural activity set up by stimulation as such, but the way the neural activity is embedded in sensorimotor dynamic.[11]

The enactive approach seeks to explain the quality of perceptual consciousness not as a neural function caused by and realized in the brain (as Searle 2004 would have it), but rather in terms of patterns and structures of skillful activity. On the enactive approach, brain, body, and world work together to make consciousness happen (Thompson and Varela 2001). Indeed, from an enactive standpoint, this is precisely what is required for an approach to count as genuinely *neurobiological*. Experience is not caused by and realized in the brain, although it depends causally on the brain. Experience is realized in the active life of the skillful animal. A neuroscience of perceptual consciousness must be an enactive neuroscience—that is, a neuroscience of embodied activity, rather than a neuroscience of brain activity.

7.8   Explanatory Limits: An Epilogue

Perceptual experience, according to the enactive approach, is an activity of exploring the environment drawing on knowledge of sensorimotor dependencies and thought. In framing the theory this way, it is easy to appreciate how the theory can be phenomenologically apt: It is intuitively plausible, for example, that the circularity of a plate becomes available in encounters with its changing perspectival shape as one moves (or would move) with respect to it (as argued in chapter 3).

This way of framing the theory, however, takes consciousness for granted. Only someone capable of mastering "patterns of sensorimotor contigency"—that is, only someone capable of keeping track of the way appearances change as he or she moves—can be capable of perceptual experience with world-presenting content. Does the enactive approach to perceptual consciousness presuppose consciousness in this way?

It was precisely in order to avoid this kind of circularity that O'Regan and I (O'Regan and Noë 2001a,b) insisted on characterizing laws of sensorimotor contingency in terms of patterns of change in sensory *stimulation* rather than in terms of changes in sensation or appearance. Only such a *physicalistic* characterization can hope to serve as a ground for a theory of consciousness. We proposed that the qualitative character of experience depended on the perceiver's practical knowledge of such patterns, and on the perceiver's ability to use this knowledge to guide thought and action. In this way, we sought to explain phenomenal consciousness in terms of forms of cognition—for instance, knowledge of patterns of sensorimotor dependence—that are, at least in principle, amenable to the sorts of explanatory practices widely deployed in cognitive science (e.g., explanation by appeal to information processing). We proposed to explain phenomenal consciousness in terms of the creature's practical knowledge of patterns of sensorimotor dependence; we took for granted that it is possible to give a noncircular and empirically adequate account of this mastery.[12]

The main problem with this strategy, I now believe, is that we purchased noncircularity and explanatory power at the expense of giving up phenomenological aptness.[13] A creature enjoys phenomenally conscious perceptual states when it has knowledge of the relevant patterns of dependence of neural activity on movement. But how can phenomenally unconscious states of this sort be the basis of phenomenal consciousness? This question remains unanswered.

We can see a way clear to a solution, I think, by placing the theory in an evolutionary setting. We can make sense of the idea that simple organisms have, if not full-fledged experience, then something like simple modes of consciousness. I don't know how to prove this, but what makes it plausible is the fact that we ourselves, in all our cognitive and phenomenological complexity, are descended from such simple organisms. It seems reasonable to hold that the conscious mind did not simply appear on the evolutionary scene, full-blown, but that it emerged gradually. In opposition to this one might argue that consciousness is not something that can come in degrees; it's all or nothing; either there is a subjective point of view, or there isn't. The matter and clutter and detail of consciousness—for example, complex visual phenomenology—may evolve, but not consciousness itself.

The enactive approach gives us the resources to frame a principled reply to this objection. To see how, let's tell an evolutionary fable. We start with the reasonable assumption that some simple lifeforms *embody* simple sensorimotor systems. A phototactic bacterium, for example, embodies a kind of sensorimotor "knowledge"; stimulation of its surfaces produce motor responses. Such a simple creature is capable of responding to stimulation; its very existence manifests an environmentally embedded sensorimotor looping. With such a maximally simple being we already have the ingredients needed for the enactment of experience. The organism is not merely a locus of mechano-chemical processes; we have a unitary being that responds and acts. Nevertheless, where the sensorimotor repertoire is rigid and simple, there is no compelling reason to attribute mind or experience. But where the sensorimotor repertoire increases in complexity, the notion that there is also primitive awareness becomes more plausible. Increasing sensorimotor complexity is at once increasing bodily and behaviorial complexity, but it is also a matter of increasing cognitive complexity, at least if we take seriously the idea that sensorimotor skills constitute a kind of knowledge. The gain in complexity can take different forms. More complex bodies mean greater degrees of freedom of movement, and so greater possible patterns of sensorimotor interaction. But there is also the possibility, investigated by Humphrey (1992), that greater sophistication includes the ability to decouple sensory stimulation from motor response. "Animals first had 'minds'," writes Humphrey, "when they first became capable of storing—and possibly recalling and reworking—action-based representations of the effects of environmental stimulation on their own bodies" (1992, 42). And he adds: "For the first time in history—the first time in fact since the universe began—certain events, namely those occurring at the surfaces of living organisms, had begun to exist as something for someone."

Whether Humphrey is right about the decoupling of sensory stimulation and motor response, the burden of the sort of account that he, and I, are putting forward is to make convincing the idea that with increasing sensorimotor complexity you get the appearance of a lifeform that embodies a measure of sensitivity to the way its own movements change the way the environment stimulates it. In this way, and with a healthy dose of hand-waving, we make plausible the idea that the emergence of perceptual consciousness in the biological world is, in effect, a matter of the emergence of cognitive agents with sensorimotor capacities. There aren't two stories: the saga of the emergence of cognitive agents, and then that of the appearance of consciousness. Consciousness and cognition are themselves aspects of the development of life.[14]

All of this is speculative, and in any case, I have only given the barest outlines of a sketch. Something like this story may be right, but even if it is, my appeal to life in this account of consciousness marks a concession. For living beings are already, by dint of being alive, *potentially conscious*. Living beings, that is, have just the sort of unity that makes it plausible to think that they might be able, for example, to "keep track" of patterns of sensorimotor covariation. A robot, in contrast, or a bit of "mere matter," seems to lack precisely that sort of unity. Who or what is it, when we are dealing with a robot, that could "notice" the way patterns of "sensory" stimulation vary as a function of movement? And in the absence of a given, unified subject, how can we hope to have explained consciousness? To take *life* for granted in an account of the emergence of consciousness may be, then, to take a *little bit* of consciousness for granted.

Perhaps the concession is not so great. First, we have certainly made progress if we can explain the whole of perceptual consciousness by presupposing, as it were, only a smidgen. You give us a spark of consciousness, we'll give you the world! Second, biology has two feet on the ground, and life is no longer the mystery that it was a hundred years ago. If we can explain consciousness (or even just perceptual consciousness) by appealing to living beings with sensorimotor and cognitive skills, then we have made progress.

A caveat is urgent, however. Biology may be on firm footing, but there is no established biological consensus on the origins of life.[15] So we may wonder whether we aren't substituting one explanatory gap for another.

At the end of this book, where do we find ourselves? I have argued that it is possible to make progress on the problems of content and qualia. The enactive approach offers a way of understanding the qualitative character of experience: Experience isn't determined by neural states set up by patterns of stimulation alone; the qualitative character of experience depends on the perceiver's mastery and exercise of sensorimotor skills. Why is an experience visual as opposed to tactile? Given that it is visual, why is it as of a sphere, rather than as of a cube? To answer these questions, you need to look not to the internal neural activations but to the way the animal's interaction with the environment is governed by skillful mastery of sensorimotor dependencies (Hurley and Noë 2003a).

Why is there any experience at all? I close with the thought that a natural philosophy of consciousness should seek answers to this question in the neighborhood of problems in biology about the nature and origins of life. It is likely that not all living things have minds; certainly there is no a priori reason to believe that only living beings could have minds. Nevertheless, for reasons I have hinted at, it may be that the problem of mind and that of life are in an important sense one. The common heart of both problems is that of understanding how "mere matter" can acquire the intrinsic unity characteristic of both the living being and the conscious point of view. Whatever we want to say about this finally, one thing is clear: For an account of consciousness to be plausible, it must be an account of consciousness as a natural phenomenon. An account of consciousness as a natural phenomenon will be a tale, not about the brain, but about our active lives.

Notes

Chapter 1 The Enactive Approach to Perception

1. What I here call the enactive approach was first presented fully in O'Regan and Noë 2001 a,b. We refer to the view as the sensorimotor contingency theory. Hurley and I, in joint work, deploy another term: the dynamic sensorimotor account. I borrow the term "enactive" from Francisco Varela and Evan Thompson (Varela, Thompson, and Rosch 1991), although I may not use it in exactly their sense. I use the term because it is apt, and to draw attention to the kinship of our view and theirs. They call "enactive" a way of thinking about the mind according to which (1) the subject of mental states is taken to be the embodied, environmentally situated animal; (2) the animal and the environment are thought of as a pair, standing in a relation of being essentially coupled and reciprocally determining; (3) perceptual and other cognitive states are thought of in terms of activity on the part of the animal and as nonrepresentational; (4) the mental life of a creature is taken to be an autonomous domain for the sort of investigation pursued within the philosophical movement known as phenomenology. My usage is as defined in the text.

2. Such skills belong to what John Searle calls the Background: the skills and capacities the possession of which makes it possible for us to carry on as we do. See Searle 1992, especially chap. 8.

3. Perspectival self-consciousness is a term of Hurley's (1998). The role of proprioception in self-actuated movement is an important theme in the work of Brian O'Shaughnessy; see his *Consciousness and the World* (2000). Whether proprioception should be thought of as a mode of *perceptual* awareness of one's body remains unresolved. O'Shaughnessy (1980) and Bermúdez (1998) argue that it ought to be. Gallagher (2003) argues that it ought not to be, citing Shoemaker (1968) and Cassam (1995) as lending support to his contention.

4. For steps in the direction of developing an enactive neuroscience of cognition and consciousness, see, for example, Hurley and Noë 2003a,b; Noë and Hurley 2003; Thompson and Varela 2001; Noë and Thompson 2004a,b; and the brief discussion

of a sensorimotor approach to the neural basis of experience in O'Regan and Noë 2001a and Noë and O'Regan 2002.

5. No doubt flies can see. What they see is (however strange this may sound) constrained by what they understand. I take up the problem of animals in chapter 6.

6. The earliest recorded instance of this medical procedure occurred in Arabia in 1020. See von Senden [1932] 1960 for a historical review of the relevant medical and philosophical literature.

7. Recently this distinction between practical and propositional knowledge has been called into question by Stanley and Williamson (2001). I discuss their criticism briefly in section 3.12.

8. Kay Toombs (1992, especially 65–68, 82–83) has investigated the way being bound in a wheelchair alters one's sense of space and agency.

9. This example is somewhat misleading. The passive kitten's visual experience is abnormal; this is explained by the fact that, harnessed as it was, the kitten was unable to acquire certain sensorimotor knowledge. It is noteworthy, however, that this passive kitten was not blind. This is not surprising. There's good reason to believe that it had sensorimotor knowledge in a substantial degree, for example, a skillful grip on the effects of eye and head movements.

10. Humphrey (1992) has developed an account of perceptual consciousness that takes as basic the sharp distinction between sensation and mere perception. Humphrey argues that sensation informs us as to what is going on with us (in or on our bodies), whereas perception is directed to the world. As Humphrey explains, this way of drawing the sensation/perception distinction is due to Reid ([1785] 1969). Crucially, on Humphrey's view, as on my own, mere sensation or feeling is not sufficient for perception.

11. It has been said that so-called blindsight—a clinical syndrome discovered by Lawrence Weiskrantz (1978)—is an example of perception without sensation. See Humphrey 1992, 86–93, for a discussion of this.

12. Hurley's 1998 book *Consciousness in Action* is an important landmark in this area. The main outlines of the enactive approach have been developed by me and O'Regan independently of Hurley; it is with pleasure and a measure of astonishment that I have come to realize to what a great extent she anticipated our work.

13. For surveys of relevant recent cognitive science, see Clark 1997, 1999; Thompson and Varela 2001; Varela, Thompson, and Rosch 1991.

14. This idea that we can forgo representation by making use of the presence of the world was perhaps first suggested by Dreyfus ([1972] 1999) and, independently, by Minsky (1985). In recent discussion, it was hit upon by Kevin O'Regan (1992) (who suggests that we let the world serve as an external memory store) and Rodney Brooks (1991) (who suggests that the world can serve as its own best model).

15. Some thinkers question whether we can really make sense of the idea of representations in the brain (e.g., Searle 1992, 2004). Others (e.g., Dennett 1981) have tried to show that talk of representation in the brain is both metaphysically harmless and scientifically useful. This is an important issue I do not pursue in this book.

16. This proposal calls to mind Strawson's treatment of the problem of "massive reduplication" (Strawson 1959, 20–23). Strawson's problem was that of securing reference when our descriptive knowledge may fail uniquely to pick out an object owing to the massive reduplication of a region of space-time. His solution was to appeal to our ability to fix reference by pointing, that is, by demonstrative reference.

17. This may be a real-world example of what Lewis (1980) called "veridical hallucination." It looks to you as if the nose is rising, when it is rising and because it is rising. Nevertheless, you don't really see it rise. This example was called to my attention by Stephen White.

18. It also rules out a stronger multiple realizability thesis according to which, say, a suitably programmed computer could be said to possess *an intelligence like ours*. The failure of the autonomy thesis *may* rule out this stronger thesis, if not in principle, then certainly in practice. This is an important topic to be pursued elsewhere. For a valuable critical discussion of the multiple realizability thesis, see Shapiro 2000.

19. Are TVSS experiences really *visual*? Block (2003) has pressed this question. I take it up in sections 3.10 and 3.11. Whatever TVSS experiences are like, they are not like the experiences of tickles on the skin. This is true despite the fact that one can direct one's attention to tickles on the skin that accompany tactile vision (as Bach-y-Rita [1996] notes).

20. Hurley (1998, especially chap. 10) offers the ingredients for a different sort of response to this worry about behaviorism. She argues that behaviorism makes the mistake of thinking of action as a simple effect of perception; the behaviorist ignores feedback from output to input. Behaviorism, as such, is a "linear or one-way view of the primary causal flows" (420). As she emphasizes, and as we have sought to develop in our work together, perception and action may be related constitutively by dynamic patterns of circular input-output-input loopings.

Chapter 2   Pictures in Mind

1. Wittgenstein discusses Mach's illustration (figure 2.1) in *Philosophical Remarks* ([1930] 1975, 267). According to Wittgenstein, Mach's drawing reveals a confusion of phenomenological (or visual) and physical modes of representation. Mach attempts to depict his experience, but he ends up depicting his room as perceived from a certain vantage point. Wittgenstein concludes that it is not possible to make a picture of the visual field. It would be a worthwhile exercise to study the different ways in which Mach's picture is unsatisfactory as a characterization of what

the seeing of the room is like. One obvious problem, noted by Wittgenstein, is that the indeterminacy of the periphery of the visual field is depicted, in Mach's picture, by a fading-to-white.

2. See Murakami and Cavanagh 2001 and Bridgeman, van der Hejiden, and Velichkovsky 1994 for detailed discussions of this phenomenon.

3. See the introduction to Noë and Thompson 2002 for more on the "orthodox conception" in the theory of vision.

4. Strictly speaking, we need to distinguish the idea that vision is a process whereby a gap-free *picture* is produced from the idea that vision is a process whereby a *representation* of the environment is produced. Importantly, there are nonpictorial (digital, symbolic) kinds of representations. Marr thought vision begins with the retinal picture. He thought of the retinal picture as an array of intensities corresponding to points of light. Although Marr believed that vision is in this way a process whereby a discontinuous picture was transformed into a detailed representation of the environment, he did not think that this resulting higher-level representation was itself pictorial; rather he thought it would be symbolic. In the text, I cast the filling-in argument as an argument for a process whereby a *picture* in the head is produced. Certainly, if we make the assumption that the higher-level representation of what is perceived is *non*pictorial (if it is symbolic, or digital), then it is becomes less clear why there should be need of *filling in*. The "filling-in" metaphor seems to presuppose that you have a continuous, picture-like representation with a gap that needs filling in. This is not logically required, however; there could be a symbolic version of the filling-in problem.

5. Lindberg (1976, 164) notes that although Leonardo in several places compares the eye to a camera obscura, he in no place compares the retina to a screen onto which images are projected. Leonardo did, however, feel it was necessary to postulate an optical process whereby inverted retinal projections were *re*inverted. This suggests that he at least tacitly assumed that the spatial properties of the retinal picture determine the spatial properties of the perceived world. For a related discussion, see Hyman 1989, 149.

6. This may have been the first time in history that anyone *actually* saw a retinal picture.

7. In what follows, I rely on Lindberg 1976, on Hyman 1989, and on presentations made by A. I. Sabra in his seminar on the history of theories of vision at Harvard University (1993–1994).

8. See Lindberg 1976, 11–17, for more on Euclid's and Ptolemy's views including detailed bibliographic references. Euclid's theory of vision is laid out in his *Optica*. Ptolemy's own ideas are laid out in a work of the same name.

9. Lindberg (1976, 11–17) makes this claim.

10. The most important texts on vision in Aristotle are *De Sensu* 2 and 3 and *De Anima* II.7 and II.12. See Aristotle 1984a,b.

11. Al-Kindi's theory of vision is laid out in his *De Aspectibus* (published in Björnbo, Anthon, and Vogl 1912). It is described in detail in Lindberg 1976, 18–32.

12. Alhazen was prolific. For a detailed description of the extant works on optics, see Lindberg 1976 and Sabra 1989.

13. According to Alhazen, objects reflect light in every direction, and every point on the surface of the eye receives light from every point in space. Each point on the eye, then, at least in a mathematical sense, is the image every point in the environment. Alhazen then proposed that the only images that play a role in generating perception are those produced by rays of light striking the surface of the eye at a 90 degree angle. See Sabra 1989 and Lindberg 1976 for a detailed introduction to these ideas.

14. This solution to the problem raises a problem of its own, however. Whatever the angle from which one sees the plate, one can see that the plate is circular. Only in exceptional circumstances would one say it looks elliptical. How can the theory of Alhazen (or indeed that of Kepler) account for perceptual constancy? I return to this topic in chapters 3 and 5.

15. For a survey of Kepler's work on vision, see Lindberg 1976, 178–208.

16. Kepler left no drawing to illustrate his conception, as noted by Lindberg 1976, 200.

17. Kepler wrote: "Indeed, I tortured myself for a long time in order to show that the cones intersecting when they pass through the aperture of the uvea intersect again behind the crystalline humour in the middle of the vitreous humour, so that another inversion is produced before they reach the retina" (qtd. in Hyman 1989, 185). The Aristotelians, it should be mentioned, were also puzzled by the question of how we have *one* visual impression despite the fact that we have two eyes.

18. This image is taken from Wade 1998, 323. For references, see Wade 1998 and Lindberg 1976.

19. Descartes wrote: "I would have you consider light as nothing else, in bodies that we call luminous, than a certain movement or action, very rapid and very lively, which passes toward our eyes through the medium of the air and other transparent bodies, in the same manner that the movement or resistance of the bodies that this blind man encounters is transmitted to his hand through the medium of his stick" ([1637] 1965, 67). This passage illustrates that Descartes' account is more thoroughly mechanistic than Kepler's. For this reason, a case can be made for regarding Descartes and not Kepler as the founder of the modern (as opposed to medieval)

study of vision. John Hyman (1989) has developed this idea. It's worth keeping in mind, however, that Descartes' account of perception relies rather heavily on a non-mechanistic theory of sensation, images, and judgment. See, for example, Descartes [1641] 1988b, 294 ("The Sixth Set of Objections").

20. The problematic homunculus reasoning does not depend on the appeal to pictures. The same problem could be raised about any kind of internal representation (whether pictorial or not). Descartes' point, in such a context, would be that internal representations cannot play a causal role in vision qua representations with intentional content, for that would presuppose an agent inside the head (as it were) who can understand them. It's worth noting that many cognitive scientists believe that the appeal to internal homunculi can be "discharged" by means of functional analysis in the case of nonpictorial representations (see Dennett [1978] 1981).

21. Whether there is evidence supporting filling in is a tricky question. In part this is because it is difficult to disentangle the problematic filling-in reasoning ("there must be filling in") from less freighted experimental work. Having said this, there is some striking evidence in favor of filling in. I mention only three bits of evidence here. (1) Murakami (1995) has shown that there is intraocular transfer of motion after effects from filled-in motion at the blind spot; (2) Paradiso and Nakayama (1991) showed that masking can affect the temporal dynamics of filling in; (3) Shimojo, Kamitani, and Nishida (2001) have shown that there are after-images of illusory (filled-in) surfaces. Each of these experiments can be interpreted to show *not merely* that subjects report a filled-in content (as it were) but that the filling-in process itself is critical. In this way these studies respond to Dennett's challenge that "the way to test my hypothesis that the brain does not bother filling-in the 'evidence' for its conclusion is to see if there are any effects that depend on the brain's having represented the *step*, rather than just the *conclusion* . . . The detail would not just *seem* to be there; it would have to be there to explain some effect" (1993, 208). For a detailed discussion of these issues, see Pessoa, Thompson, and Noë 1998.

22. This paragraph borrows from Noë, Pessoa, and Thompson 2000.

23. Bruce Bridgeman performs this experiment with his students in Psychology 1 at UC Santa Cruz each year. Students laugh at the unexpected blindness of the subjects.

24. O'Regan is now careful to avoid this conclusion.

25. In addition to the authors cited in chapter 1, note 14, Clark (1997) has developed this idea.

26. O'Regan, Rensink, and Clark 1996, 1999; Rensink, O'Regan, and Clark 1997, 2000; Simons and Levin 1998.

27. See Simons et al. 2002; Angelone, Levin, and Simons 2003; Levin et al. 2002; Mitroff, Simons, and Levin forthcoming.

28. The term was introduced by Mack and Rock. A detailed study of the phenomenon is contained in their book (1998). For further discussion, in connection with the themes of this chapter, see Noë and O'Regan 2000.

29. As mentioned earlier, O'Regan no longer defends the grand illusion hypothesis. See, for example, O'Regan and Noë 2001a,b.

30. See Pessoa, Thompson, and Noë (1998); Thompson, Noë, and Pessoa (1999); and Noë, Pessoa, and Thompson (2000) for more on Dennett's thought in this area.

31. As argued in Noë, Pessoa, and Thompson 2000 and in Noë 2002c.

32. See Thompson, Noë, and Pessoa 1999 for further development of this line of criticism.

33. Blackmore writes: "When we open our eyes and look around it seems as though we are experiencing a rich and ever-changing picture of the world" (2002, 19). This echoes her 1995 collaboration (Blackmore et al. 1995). However, she has moved much closer to my view. In the same paper, Blackmore writes: "There is no stable, rich visual representation in our minds that could be the contents of the stream of consciousness . . . Yet it seems there is, doesn't it? Well, does it? . . . I suggest we all need to look again—and look very hard, with persistence and practice" (2002, 23). This suggests she now believes that a more careful reflection on the character of our experience (phenomenology) does not support the claim that it seems to us as if all the detail is in consciousness.

34. For more on this line of criticism, see Noë, Pessoa, and Thompson 2000; Noë and O'Regan 2000; and O'Regan and Noë 2001a; Noë 2002c; Noë 2005.

35. Levin (2002) has shown experimentally that perceivers are consistently overconfident about the degree to which they will detect visual changes. He argues that this is evidence of "a deeper metacognitive error" that he and his colleagues call change blindness blindness or CBB (Levin et al. 2000). CBB is a pervasive metacognitive error and one, he points out, with potentially great importance for matters of public policy (e.g., the assessment of eyewitness reliability, the assessment of responsibility in traffic accidents, the design of human/machine interfaces, etc.). Although Levin claims that the grand illusion is real, he is also careful to explain that people are not generally deluded about their visual experience. He certainly does not give evidence that normal perceivers are committed to anything like the Machian picture.

36. This example of the held bottle is first used by MacKay (1962, 1967, 1973). It has been used by O'Regan (1992), Clark (1997), and Noë (2001).

37. See Thompson, Noë, and Pessoa 1999 for more on this distinction.

38. I depend here on the line of argument developed in O'Regan and Noë 2001a,b; Noë and O'Regan 2000; O'Regan, Myin, and Noë forthcoming. In these papers,

however, we contrast the *corporality* of sensorimotor dependences with their *alerting capacity*. Corporality refers precisely to what I, in the text, call movement dependence. However, "alerting capacity" does not refer to object dependence (i.e., to the way object movement produces sensory change), but rather to the way "incoming sensory stimulation peremptorily influences attention." O'Regan, to whom this idea is due, has proposed that we construct a "phenomenal plot," in which all qualia can be plotted in Cartesian coordinates, where the abscissa is degree of corporality and the ordinate is degree of alerting capacity. See O'Regan, Myin, and Noë forthcoming. We have sought to develop these ideas in these papers with, to date, somewhat limited success.

39. In 3.12 I return to the question of the nature of sensorimotor knowledge.

40. Pessoa, Thompson, and Noë (1998) and Thompson, Noë, and Pessoa (1999) also took for granted that it is correct to say, at the personal level, that we experience a filled-in percept in the sense that we take ourselves to have the experience that we would have if the line were gap-free even though it is not.

41. This mistake comes out clearly in Palmer's attempt (1999a, 617) to represent graphically the experience of a filled-in line in the same way as he represents the experience of an unbroken line. In general, from the fact that it looks as if the line is unbroken (when the break in the line falls on the blind spot), it does not follow that the perceptual experience as of a broken line whose break falls on the blind spot and an unbroken line are identical.

42. Two other examples: (1) Shimojo has recently demonstrated that you will experience a single flash of light as a double flash, if, when the flash occurs, there is a double click. The sound induces a visual illusion. As Shimojo recognizes (in personal communication), although it is true that the double click produces the illusion of a double flash, the illusory double flash doesn't look the same as an actual double flash. (2) When discrepant images are projected independently to each eye, subjects experience so-called binocular rivalry. This phenomenon is usually described as, for example, the experience of the alternation of the two images. As in the other cases we have considered, however, the experience of the alternation of the two images is not identical, qualitatively, to the experience of the corresponding alternation of distal stimuli (except perhaps in unusual circumstances). There are other differences as well. In binocular rivalry there is the sense that the alternation is endogenously produced. In addition, instead of experiencing a simple alternation, subjects usually experience a complex series of variations where the two images form extremes.

43. Grice spoke of the *diaphonous* quality of perceptual experience. As Grice writes: "Such experiences . . . as seeing and feeling seem to be, as it were, diaphanous: if we were asked to pay close attention, on a given occasion, to our seeing or feeling as distinct from what was being seen or felt, we should not know how to proceed; and

the attempt to describe the differences between seeing and feeling seems to dissolve into a description of what we see and what we feel" (1962, 144). Transparency has been much discussed in recent philosophical writing about experience. Recently several writers—among them, Harman, Tye, and Dretske—have defended *representationism*, that is, the view that the qualitative character of experience is exhausted by its representational content. For representationists, it is important that a description of the experience is, of necessity, a description of what the experience represents. See Stoljar (forthcoming) for an excellent critical discussion and survey of ideas about the transparency of experience. See also Harman 1990; Dretske 1995; Tye 2000, chap. 3; Martin 2002; and Siewert (2004).

Chapter 3   Enacting Content

1. To see something *as* round is, in philosophical usage, to see it as falling under the concept *round*. In chapter 6 I turn to the question of the role of concepts in perception and perceptual consciousness.

2. Peacocke (1983) discusses this example, as do I in Noë 2002a.

3. For discussion of this point, see Hacker 1987.

4. For descriptions of Ames's demonstrations, see Ittelson 1952 and Gregory [1966] 1997, 177–181.

5. See Hyman 1989 for a similar account. See also my discussion in Noë 2002a. In Noë 2002a, I referred to perspectival properties as occlusion properties (or O-properties), following Hyman 1989.

6. P-properties are also objective according to Frege's criterion: "What is objective . . . is what is subject to laws, what can be conceived and judged, what is expressible in words. What is purely intuitable is not communicable" ([1884] 1950, 35).

7. I consider a perspectival account of color in chapter 4.

8. Wollheim ([1968] 1980, 205–226) has emphasized the idea of *seeing in*. We see an object *in* a picture, for example. I call on a similar idea in the text. Just as it is the case that you see a picture, and, in seeing the picture, you see what the picture depicts (and so in that sense see the depicted item in the picture), so I want to suggest that we see the elliptical perspectival properties and, in seeing them, we see the plate's circularity (and so in that sense see the circularity in the elliptical perspectival properties). However, I would not want to suggest that seeing appearances is like seeing pictures, or that perspectival properties *depict* nonperspectival properties. This was certainly not Wollheim's view.

9. I discuss other modalities later in this chapter (section 3.10) and also in chapter 4 (4.10).

10. For philosophical discussion of the idea of egocentric space, see Campbell 1994; Evans 1982, 1985, essay 13 (reprinted in Noë and Thompson 2002).

11. Thanks to Bence Nanay for pressing me to clarify my position in relation to the "perception is for action" view.

12. For a discussion of Harris's treatment of inverting goggles, see Hurley 1998.

13. Two papers challenging spectrum inversion are Campbell 1993 and Byrne and Hilbert 1997.

14. Pettit (2003b) has recently attempted to argue that experience of color may be much more like experience of motion and space than philosophers have been inclined to think. He is guided by the thought that if inversion is incoherent in the spatial case, perhaps it's incoherent in the color case too.

15. As suggested by Botvinick and Cohen (1998). Subjects were "seated with their left arm resting upon a small table. A standing screen was positioned beside the arm to hide it from the subject's view and a life-sized rubber model of a left hand and arm was placed on the table directly in front of the subject. The subject sat with eyes fixed on the artificial hand while we used two small paintbrushes to stroke the rubber hand and the subject's hidden hand, synchronizing the timing of the brushing as closely as possible" (Botvinik and Cohen 1998, 756). After a short interval, subjects have the distinct and unmistakable feeling that they sense the stroking and tapping in the visible rubber hand and not in the hand that is in fact being touched. Further tests show that if you then ask subjects with closed eyes to point to the left hand with the hidden hand, their pointings, after experience of the illusion, are displaced toward the rubber hand. Botvinik and Cohen suggest that this experiment lends support to the idea that our sense of our body as our own depends on its differentiation from other objects thanks to "its participation in specific forms of intermodal correlation" (756). The idea is that the body image is a model produced by the brain to organize information received from the different senses. But strikingly, it only takes a few tricks to force the brain to alter the model (Ramachandran and Blakeslee 1998). Whether this is right or not, what these strange experiments seem to show is the importance, for haptic perception, not just of touch, but of what we see, and of what we understand to be going on. The establishment of a visual correlation is enough, it seems, to produce felt sensation. (The title of Botvinick and Cohen's article is "Rubber hands 'feel' touch that eyes see.")

16. This point was called to my attention by Susan Hurley. I am indebted to her for discussion of Harris's treatment of this issue.

17. Among those who discussed this question are the following: John Locke, Gottfried Wilhelm Leibniz, George Berkeley, Julien Offray de La Mettrie, Denis Diderot, Etienne Bonnot de Condillac, John Stuart Mill, Hermann Ludwig Ferdinand von Helmholtz, William James, M. von Senden, Donald Hebb, Gareth Evans, R. L. Gregory, and Oliver Sacks.

18. They write: "Where Gibson speaks of directly perceiving features of the layout in consequence of picking up features of the light, the Establishment theory speaks of perceiving features of the layout in consequence of transducing features of the light. Thus far, the differences are merely terminological. The important fact is the agreement that the subject's epistemic relation to the structure of the light is different from his epistemic relation to the layout of the environment, and that the former relation is causally dependent on the latter" (Fodor and Pylyshyn 1981, 165).

19. Fodor and Pylyshyn argue that for Gibson the fact that the light contains information about the layout is the result of the fact that there is a causally mediated correlation between the layout and the light. But then "contains information" is a symmetric relation. The layout can with just as much right be said to contain information about the light.

20. A similar view is developed by von Senden ([1932] 1960) and by Jonas (1966).

21. Keeley (2001) proposes that the vomeronasal system is a sensory modality that lacks qualia, and he offers this as a counterexample to the view that the senses can be individuated by their different qualia. I agree, but for different reasons, that the senses cannot be individuated in terms of qualia.

22. Preliminary work (a submitted report by R. Kuppers et al., cited in Block 2003) suggests there may in fact be occipital lobe activity in TVSS as well.

23. I am grateful to Christopher Peacocke (personal communication) for this criticism.

24. I am grateful to Benj Hellie for discussion of this point.

25. Thanks to Dave Chalmers for discussion of this.

Chapter 4   Colors Enacted

1. Alan Gilchrist has shown this; a demonstration—*Bright Black*—based on his work has been on display at the San Francisco Exploratorium, where I saw it.

2. Sean Kelly (2001) locates the problem in a somewhat different place than Peacocke (1983, 2001). Kelly proposes that there is a qualitative difference between our experience of the two parts of the wall, and he grants that this is a difference in the representational content of our experience, a difference in how the experience presents the wall as being. But he doubts that this difference is a difference in *color* (and, in particular, that it is a difference that makes a difference to our use of color concepts). In personal communication, he has urged that although it is true that we can see the wall as varied in color across its surface, and that we can see it as uniform in color, we can't have these experiences at the same time. Either we attend to the uniformity of the underlying color, or to its nonuniformity, but we can't do both simultaneously. He proposes that we think of the way color appearance varies as an

effect of background context. When we experience the variability of the wall's surface color, we are experiencing the different ways the single color looks as lighting
varies. I am sympathetic to the idea that the way a color looks changes as lighting
conditions change—and so with the idea that not every change in lighting is a
change in color. I am also sympathetic to the idea that one cannot attend, simula-
taneously, to the constancy and the variability of color. Nevertheless, Kelly's position seems to explain away the problem of presence and constancy without
explaining it. When I look at my wall now I see its uniform color *in* the variations
of its apparent color across the surface. Experienced perceivers understand that
colors, like 3-D objects, have aspects, and they understand, implicitly, that
changes (in position, in lighting) produce changes in the way things look with
respect to color.

3. In O'Regan and Noë 2001a, we argue that the two kinds of sensorimotor rules
correspond to sensation and perception, respectively.

4. Block expresses a similar thought. He writes: "You ask: What is it that philosophers have called qualitative states? I answer, only half in jest: As Louis Armstrong
said when asked what Jazz is, 'If you got to ask, you ain't never gonna get to know'"
(1978, 281).

5. Alternatively, one might say that this sort of account explains what it could mean
to say that the bee, the normal human, and the prosthetic perceiver all occupy the
same point of view.

6. Byrne and Hilbert (2003, sec. 2.5) criticize Thompson's ecological approach
(1995) on the grounds that it is, in effect, a version of the traditional dispositionalism. But Thompson's approach, and that developed here, differs from the traditional dispositional theory in three major ways. First, according to the traditional
view, colors are relations between surfaces, say, and perceivers (or perceivers'
minds). On the ecological view they are relations between surfaces and the environment. Second, the traditional view cashes out the idea that colors are phenomenal in terms of the idea that they are sensations. The ecological view, in
contrast, treats them as phenomenal in the sense of appearances (Thompson
1995). (On my view, appearances are real.) Third, according to the ecological
approach, colors are properties of the world—they are out there—but they are not
physical properties as such, even though they are natural properties. They are
properties of the environment.

7. Kohler's work on these colored lenses is of importance for the philosophical theory of color. Very few philosophers have discussed it. Exceptions are Hurley 1998,
O'Regan and Noë 2001a, and Pettit 2003a.

8. Justin Broackes (1992) offers an observation that might lead one to be optimistic
about prospects for enabling color experience in the blind. He notes that subjects

with normal dichromatic (e.g., red-green) color blindness are typically able visually to track and sift reds and greens. What do we track when we track color? What we track are patterns of variation under movement and environmental changes. Dichromacy, it turns out, only affects one's ability thus to track changes in a very limited range of cases.

Chapter 5   Perspective in Content

1. This general line of objection has been advanced by Stephen White (personal communication).

2. As I discuss in chapter 3, note 8, Wollheim's notion of "seeing in" is helpful here. When you see a man in a picture, you see both the picture *and* the man at once.

3. This is true of the sensory modalities of hearing and touch as well, although in the case of touch, the grip of the term "perspectival" loosens.

4. Mirrors may provide a further example. You see the police in the rearview mirror, but in seeing them, you mis-experience their location relative to you. We rarely notice the perspectival nonveridicality in cases such as this, because they are so familiar. In other cases, this is more apparent. For example, it is rather difficult (for some of us at least) to *see*, of the car in the mirror, which side is the driver's side. Thanks to Casey O'Callahan for this example.

5. I take it that it matters that you are watching the game on TV "live," namely, in real time. The security guard, for example, really watches (and sees) the crowd on closed-circuit monitors. Exactly what the role of time is in perceptual experience is tricky. Can you see the stars in the sky, even though they may no longer exist?

6. As we have seen in previous chapters, recent work on prosthetic perception in the perceptual and neural sciences shows that these are not idle points. See, for example, Bach-y-Rita 1996.

7. Actually, the nonperceptuality of this case may have been overdetermined. Not only is there a failure of perceptual dependence, but it is hard to imagine that factual dependence could be really maintained by the fiddlings of a surgeon. We naturally suppose that it won't be the case that experience changes with every little visible change in how things are around you. As is frequently the case in philosophy, our intuitions are driven by the way in which cases are *under*described.

8. In the natural world, however, it may be that the only way to preserve the right kinds of dependence relations between experience and the world is by the standard, biologically realized ways with which we are familiar. From a certain standpoint, artificial perceptual systems are very much like biological ones. Importantly,

the inadequacy of such systems is in direct proportion to the degree to which they are different from ordinary, biological systems.

9. I take up this question in Noë 2001b. In this paper I argue that (some) art can make a contribution to a science of consciousness by making a contribution to phenomenology. Merleau-Ponty believed something similar: He held that art was phenomenologically prior to science (Merleau-Ponty 1964; Priest 1998, 206). According to Merleau-Ponty, painters can explore the visible, and so explore the world as experienced. Painting thus depends on and illuminates the fact that we are embodied and "in the world." Merleau-Ponty writes: "We cannot imagine how a mind could paint. It is by lending his body to the world that the artist changes the world into paintings. To understand these transubstantiations we must go back to the working, actual body—not the body as a chunk of space or a bundle of functions but that body which is an intertwining of vision and movement" (1964, 162; qtd. in Priest 1998, 210, Priest's translation).

10. Pinker's view may be an instance of what Wollheim has called the resemblance view of pictoriality. See Wollheim 1998 for a discussion of this. He cites Peacocke 1987 and Budd 1993 as sophisticated examples of this sort of approach.

11. The account of pictoriality I sketch here is compatible with Wollheim's "seeing-in" theory of representation. I support Wollheim's idea of the twofoldedness of our experience of the picture and that which it represents. We can see both simultaneously. This is how things are in perception more generally; we see how things appear and we see how things are. Perceptual consciousness is folded in this way. See Wollheim 1998 and [1968] 1980.

Chapter 6   Thought in Experience

1. Putnam (1992, 1999) uses this term "proto-concept" in connection with animal cognitive capacities.

2. I take it that Wittgenstein's claim (1953, sec. 201) that there is a way of following a rule that does not depend on a further act of interpretation expresses the thought that sometimes our grasp of the application of a concept is more immediate than this.

3. Some might say that basic concepts such as *red* and *valid* are concepts that are applied on the basis of nonconceptual grounds. To understand such a concept is just to apply it in an appropriate condition, even though one has no concept of the condition itself. This has been argued by Peacocke (1992). But this seems doubtful. The point is not that such concepts get applied on nonconceptual grounds, but that they are not applied on the basis of grounds at all. Explanation, as Wittgenstein said, comes to an end.

4. This is compatible with its being the case that one can see an anteater even

though one lacks the concept of an anteater. Following Dretkse (1993), we can distinguish propositional seeing (seeing *that* such and such is the case), from object seeing (seeing *x*). If I am right that perceptual experience is conceptual, then it is always the case that whenever one undergoes an experience of seeing *x*, one has a visual experience that can be described as having propositional (and so conceptual) content.

5. Commitment to this Machian idea may be implicated by Peacocke's conception of scenario content (Peacocke 1992). The scenario content of a perceptual experience is said to be the way of filling out the space around the individual such that the experience is veridical. Scenario content is nonconceptual, according to this view, because the perceiver need not, in order to have the experience, possess the concepts needed to capture in thought the ways of filling out the space that would make the experience veridical. The problem is, we do not in fact experience all the filled-out detail in the scene all at once. It can't be right to suggest that such a filled-out space gives the *content of what is experienced*.

6. One of the problems with Mach's picture of the visual field (as noticed by Wittgenstein) is that Mach's drawing misrepresents the nature of the indeterminacy. He depicts the extreme periphery of the visual field as faded-to-white, whereas the actually periphery is experienced as continuous with what is in central focus.

Chapter 7   Brain in Mind

1. It is precisely in response to the need to make intelligible the relation between the neural system and the experience that many scientists implictly rely on the idea that there must be a kind of correspondence or "explanatory isomorphism" between properties of the substrate and properties of the resulting experience, as discussed in Noë and Thompson (2004a,b) and Pessoa, Thompson, and Noë (1998). If there were no relation, however abstract, beyond brute correlation, the dependence of experience on a neural substrate would remain a mystery. One way to capture the argument in the text would be by saying that we now lack any reason *beyond mere correlation* to think that a neural system could be the substrate of (the sufficient basis for) an experience.

2. This topic forms the main focus of ongoing joint work by me and Susan Hurley. I draw on our joint work in this chapter.

3. There is empirical work to support this claim. Stephen LaBerge (personal communication) has argued that his work with lucid dreamers supports this finding.

4. See chapter 1, note 14, for sources for this important idea.

5. Vehicle externalism about perceptual experience is a minority position. With the exception of Hurley (1998) and Rowlands (2002, 2003), I don't know any philoso-

phers who take it seriously. Hurley and I are now writing a book in which we develop the argument further.

6. I consider this possibility in Noë 2001. Thanks to Bence Nanay for pressing its importance in the present context.

7. Stephen White has raised this objection to me in personal communication. I have also benefitted from discussion of this topic with Bert Dreyfus and John Searle.

8. Why don't I concede that if it were true that neural duplicates would always agree in their experience, regardless of the environment, then the neural sufficiency thesis is out-and-out established? Because this possibility still leaves open that neural systems might require *some* non-neural context in order to operate correctly.

9. General support for the enactive approach in neuroscience comes from Alvaro Pascual-Leone. He has has advanced the theory of the metamodal brain (Pascual-Leone and Hamilton 2001). Pascual-Leone questions the very identification of sensory processing in one modality or another with patterns of activity in brain regions. There aren't modality-specific regions of the brain. For example, normal touch has been shown to depend on neural activity in "visual" cortex.

10. When they are thus integrated—as when patients with phantoms make use of Ramachandran's "mirror-box" therapy—the experience of referred sensation to the missing limb lessens. See Ramachandran and Blakeslee 1998, 47ff.

11. Synesthesia provides a similar case. See Hurley and Noë 2003a and Noë and Hurley 2003. We are continuing work on this topic. Synesthesia and phantom limb cases are examples of what we call cortical dominance; that is, in these cases neural structures preserve their previous qualitative expression in the face of novel inputs. Cases of plasticity such as those mentioned in the text (TVSS, visual-to-auditory rerouting in ferrets, the blind readers of Braille) are examples of what we call "cortical deference"; in these cases, a cortical area changes its qualitative expression to accommodate a nonstandard pattern of input.

12. When Clark and Toribio (2001) challenged us to admit that on our view a Ping-Pong-playing robot would be visually conscious, we replied that a Ping-Pong-playing robot would be perceptually conscious only if it could be demonstrated to have real *knowledge* (genuine mastery) of the relevant visual sensorimotor contingencies. Nothing in our view committed us to saying that the robot would be perceptually conscious. All we committed ourself to is the possibility that such a robot could be perceptually conscious *if* it acquired the relevant practical skills. Give us a cognitive agent, and we'll show you how to give it consciousness.

13. There is a second problem as well. It may be that we underestimated the difficulty of giving an account of cognition.

14. Evan Thompson has influenced my thinking about these issues. In his book *Radical Embodiment* (forthcoming), he proposes what he calls the "mind-life continuity hypothesis."

15. This is not a controversial statement. Dawkins (1976), Kauffman (1995), and Dennett (1995), for example, all acknowledge that although we have ideas about how life may have begun, we haven't figured out how it did begin.

Works Cited

Albers, J. 1963. *Interaction of Color*. New Haven, CT: Yale University Press.

Angelone, B. L., D. T. Levin, and D. J. Simons. 2003. The roles of representation and comparison failures in change blindness. *Perception* 32: 947–962.

Anscombe, G. E. M. 1965. The intentional of sensation: A grammatical feature. In *Metaphysics and the Philosophy of Mind: Collected Philosophical Papers,* vol. III, 3–20. Oxford: Blackwell.

Arbib, M. A. 1989. *The Metaphorical Brain 2: Neural Networks and Beyond*. New York: Wiley.

Aristotle. 1984a. *De Anima*. In *The Complete Works of Aristotle: The Revised Oxford Translation*. Oxford: Oxford University Press.

Aristotle. 1984b. *De Sensu*. In *The Complete Works of Aristotle: The Revised Oxford Translation*. Oxford: Oxford University Press.

Armstrong, D. M. 1961. *Perception and the Physical World*. London: Routledge & Kegan Paul.

Armstrong, D. M. 1968. *A Materialist Theory of Mind*. London: Routledge & Kegan Paul.

Austin, J. L. 1962. *Sense and Sensibilia*. Oxford: Clarendon Press.

Ayer, A. J. 1955. *The Foundations of Empirical Knowledge*. London: Macmillan.

Ayer, A. J. 1973. *The Central Questions of Philosophy*. New York: Holt, Rinehart, Winston.

Bach-y-Rita, P. 1972. *Brain Mechanisms in Sensory Substitution*. New York: Academic Press.

Bach-y-Rita, P. 1983. Tactile vision substitution: Past and future. *International Journal of Neuroscience* 19, nos. 1–4: 29–36.

Bach-y-Rita, P. 1984. The relationship between motor processes and cognition in tactile vision substitution. In *Cognition and Motor Processes,* ed. A. F. Sanders and W. Prinz, 150–159. Berlin: Springer.

Bach-y-Rita, P. 1996. Substitution sensorielle et qualia [Sensory substitution and qualia]. In *Perception et Intermodalité,* ed. J. Proust, 81–100. Paris: Presses Universitaires de France. Reprinted in English translation in *Vision and Mind: Selected Readings in the Philosophy of Perception,* ed. A. Noë and E. Thompson, 497–514. Cambridge, MA: The MIT Press, 2002.

Bach-y-Rita, P., and S. Kercel. 2002. Sensory substitution and augmentation: Incorporating humans-in-the-loop. *Intellectica* 2, no. 35: 287–297.

Ballard, D. H. 1991. Animate vision. *Artificial Intelligence* 48: 57–86.

Ballard, D. H. 1996. On the function of visual representation. In *Perception: Volume 5, Vancouver Studies in Cognitive Science,* ed. Kathleen Akins, 111–131. New York: Oxford University Press. Reprinted in *Vision and Mind: Selected Readings in the Philosophy of Perception,* ed. A. Noë and E. Thompson, 459–479. Cambridge, MA: The MIT Press, 2002.

Ballard, D. H. 2002. Our perception of the world has to be an illusion. *Journal of Consciousness Studies* 9, nos. 5–6: 54–71.

Bennett, M. R., and P. M. S. Hacker. 2001. Perception and memory in neuroscience: A conceptual analysis. *Progress in Neurobiology* 65, no. 6: 499–543.

Berkeley, G. [1709] 1975. Essay towards a new theory of vision. In *George Berkeley: Philosophical Works, including the Works on Vision,* ed. M. R. Ayers, 1–59. London and Totowa, NJ: Dent and Rowman and Littlefield.

Bermúdez, J. L. 1998. *The Paradox of Self-Consciousness.* Cambridge, MA: The MIT Press.

Berthoz, A. [1997] 2000. *The Brain's Sense of Movement.* Trans. Giselle Weiss. Cambridge, MA: Harvard University Press.

Billock, V. A., G. A. Gleason, and B. H. Tsou. 2001. Perception of forbidden colors in retinally stabilized equiluminant images: An indication of softwired color opponency? *Journal of the Optical Society of America* 18, no. 10: 2398–2403.

Björnbo, A., A. Anthon, and S. Vogl. 1912. Alkindi, Tideus und Pseudo-Euklid. Drei optische Werke. *Abhandlung zur Geschichte der mathematischen Wissenschaften* 26, pt. 3: 1–176.

Blackmore, S. J. 2002. There is no stream of consciousness. In *Is the Visual World a Grand Illusion?,* ed. A. Noë, 17–28. Thorverton, UK: Academic Imprint.

Blackmore, S. J., G. Brelstaff, K. Nelson, and T. Troscianko. 1995. Is the richness of our visual world an illusion? Transsaccadic memory for complex scenes. *Perception* 24: 1075–1081.

Block, N. 1978. Troubles with functionalism. In *Minnesota Studies in the Philosophy Science,* vol. 9, ed. C. Wade Savage, 261–325. Minneapolis: University of Minnesota Press.

Block, N. 1990. Inverted earth. In *Philosophical Perspectives 4, Action Theory and Philosophy of Mind,* ed. J. Tomberlin, 53–79. Atascadero, CA: Ridgeview.

Block, N. 2001. Behaviorism revisited. *Behavioral & Brain Sciences* 24: 977–978.

Block, N. 2003. Tactile sensation via spatial perception. *Trends in Cognitive Sciences* 7, no. 7: 285–286.

Boghossian, P. A., and D. J. Velleman. 1989. Colour as a secondary quality. *Mind* 98: 81–103.

Boghossian, P. A., and D. J. Velleman. 1991. Physicalist theory of color. *Philosophical Review* 100: 67–106.

Botvinick, M., and J. Cohen. 1998. Rubber hands 'feel' touch that eyes see [letter]. *Nature* 391, no. 6669: 756.

Boyson, S., G. Bernston, M. Hannan, and J. Cacioppo. 1996. Quantity-based inference and symbolic representation in chimpanzees (Pan troglodytes). *Journal of Experimental Psychology and Animal Behavior Processes* 22: 76–86.

Bridgeman, B. 1992. Conscious vs. unconscious processes: The case of vision. *Theory & Psychology* 2 (1): 73–88.

Bridgeman, B., A. Gemmer, T. Forsman, and V. Huemer. 2000. Properties of the sensorimotor branch of the visual system. *Vision Research* 40: 3539–3552.

Bridgeman, B., M. Kirch, and A. Sperling. 1981. Segregation of cognitive and motor aspects of visual function using induced motion. *Perception and Psychophysics* 29: 336–342.

Bridgeman, B., S. Lewis, F. Heit, and M. Nagle. 1979. Relation between the cognitive and motor-oriented systems of visual position perception. *Journal of Experimental Psychology: Human Perception and Performance* 5: 692–700.

Bridgeman, B., A. H. C. Van der Heijden, and B. M. Velichkovsky. 1994. A theory of visual stability across saccadic eye movements. *Behavioral and Brain Sciences* 17, no. 2: 247–292.

Broackes, J. 1992. The autonomy of colour. In *Reduction, Explanation and Realism,* ed. D. Charles and K. Lennon, 421–465. Oxford: Oxford University Press.

Brooks, R. A. 1991. Intelligence without reason. *Proceedings of the 12th International Joint Conference on Artificial Intelligence, Sydney, Australia* (August): 569–595.

Bruce, V., and P. R. Green. [1985] 1990. *Visual Perception: Physiology, Psychology and Ecology.* London: Lawrence Erlbaum.

Buchel, C. 1998. Functional neuroimaging studies of Braille reading: Cross-modal reorganization and its implications. *Brain* 121:1193–1194.

Buchel, C., C. Price, R. S. J. Frackowiak, and K. Friston. 1998. Different activation patterns in the visual cortex of late and congenitally blind subjects. *Brain* 121: 409–19.

Budd, M. 1993. How pictures look. In *Virtue and Taste,* ed. D. Knowles and J. Skorupsky. Oxford: Blackwell.

Byrne, A., and D. Hilbert. 1997. Colors and reflectances. In *Reading on Color, Vol.1: The Philosophy of Color,* ed. A. Byrne and D. Hilbert. Cambridge, MA: The MIT Press.

Byrne, A., and D. Hilbert. 2003. Color realism and color science. *Behavioral and Brain Sciences* 26: 3–21.

Campbell, J. 1993. A simple view of colour. In *Reality, Representation and Projection,* ed. J Haldane and C. Wright. Oxford: Oxford University Press.

Campbell, J. 1994. *Past, Space, and Self.* Cambridge, MA: The MIT Press.

Cassam, Q. 1995. Introspection and bodily self-ascription. In *The Body and the Self,* ed. J. L. Bermúdez, A. J. Marcel, and N. Eilan, 311–336. Cambridge, MA: The MIT Press, 1995.

Chalmers, D. J. 1996. *The Conscious Mind: In Search of a Fundamental Theory.* New York: Oxford University Press.

Cheney, D. L., and R. M. Seyfarth. 1990. *How Monkeys See the World.* Chicago: University of Chicago Press.

Chomsky, N. 1965. *Aspects of the Theory of Syntax.* Cambridge, MA: The MIT Press.

Chomsky, N. 1980. *Rules and Representations.* New York: Columbia University Press.

Churchland, P. S., V.S., Ramachandran, and T. J. Sejnowsky. 1994. A critique of pure vision. In *Large-Scale Neuronal Theories of the Brain,* ed. C. Koch and J. L. Davis, 23–60. Cambridge, MA: The MIT Press.

Clark, A. 1997. *Being There: Putting Brain, Body and World Together Again.* Cambridge, MA: The MIT Press.

Clark, A. 1999. An embodied cognitive science? *Trends in Cognitive Sciences* 3: 345–351.

Clark, A. 2002. Is seeing all it seems?: Action, reason and the grand illusion. *Journal of Consciousness Studies* 9, nos. 5–6: 181–202.

Clark, A., and D. J. Chalmers. 1998. The extended mind. *Analysis* 58: 10–23.

Clark, A., and J. Toribio. 2001. Sensorimotor chauvinism? *Behavioral and Brain Sciences* 24: 5, 979–981.

Clark, J. J. 2002. Asymmetries in ecological and sensorimotor laws: Towards a theory of subjective experience. Paper presented at the 3rd Workshop on the Genesis of the Notion of Space in Machines and Humans, Paris, France, October. Available at http://www.cim.mcgill.ca/~clark/publications.html.

Clarke, T. 1965. Seeing surfaces and physical objects. In *Philosophy in America*, ed. M. Black, 98–114. Ithaca: Cornell University Press.

Cohen, L. G., P. Celnik, A. Pascual-Leone, B. Corwell, L. Faiz, J. Dambrosia, M. Honda, N. Sadato, C. Gerloff, M. D. Catala, and M. Hallett. 1997. Functional relevance of cross-modal plasticity in blind humans. *Nature* 389: 180–183.

Cole, J. 1991 *Pride and the Daily Marathon*. London: Duckworth.

Cole, J. 2004. *Still Lives: Narratives in Spinal Cord Injury*. Cambridge, MA: The MIT Press.

Cosmides, L. 1989. The logic of social exchange: Has natural selection shaped how humans reason? Studies with the Wason Selection Task. *Cognition* 31: 187–276.

Cotterill, R. M. J. 1995. On the unity of conscious experience. *Journal of Consciousness Studies* 2, no. 4: 290–312.

Cotterill, R. M. J. 2001. Cooperation of the basal ganglia, cerebellum, sensory cerebrum and hippocampus: Possible implications for cognition, consciousness, intelligence and creativity. *Progress in Neurobiology* 64(1): 1–33.

Crane, H., and T. P. Piantinida. 1983. On seeing reddish green and yellowish blue. *Science* 221: 1078–1080.

Crane, T. 1992. The nonconceptual content of experience. In *The Contents of Experience*, ed. Tim Crane, 136–157. Cambridge: Cambridge University Press.

Crick, F., and C. Koch. 2003. A framework for consciousness. *Nature Neuroscience* 6, no. 2: 119–126.

Cussins, A. 2003. Experience, thought and activity. In *Essays on Nonconceptual Content*, ed. Y. Gunther, 133–163. Cambridge, MA: The MIT Press.

Damasio, A. R. 1994. *Descartes' Error: Emotion, Reason and the Human Brain*. New York: Avon Books.

Davidson, D. 1982. Rational animals. *Dialectica* 36: 318–327.

Dawkins, R. 1976. *The Selfish Gene*. New York: Oxford University Press.

Dennett, D. C. 1969. *Content and Consciousness*. London: Routledge & Kegan Paul.

Dennett, D. C. [1978] 1981. Artificial intelligence as philosophy and as psychology. In *Brainstorms*. Cambridge, MA: The MIT Press.

Dennett, D. C. 1981. *Brainstorms*. Cambridge, MA: The MIT Press.

Dennett, D. C. [1981] 1987. Three kinds of intentional psychology. In *Reduction, Time and Reality*, ed. R. Healey, 37–61. Cambridge: Cambridge University Press. Reprinted in *The Intentional Stance*, 43–68. Cambridge, MA: The MIT Press.

Dennett, D. C. 1987. *The Intentional Stance*. Cambridge, MA: MIT Press.

Dennett, D. C. 1991. *Consciousness Explained*. Boston: Little, Brown.

Dennett, D. C. 1993. Back from the drawing board. In *Dennett and His Critics*, ed. B. Dahlbom, 203–235. Oxford: Basil Blackwell.

Dennett, D. C. 1995 *Darwin's Dangerous Idea*. New York: Touchstone Books.

Dennett, D. C. 2001. Surprise, surprise. *Behavioral & Brain Sciences* 24: 982.

Dennett, D. C. 2002. How could I be wrong? How wrong could I be? In *Is the Visual World a Grand Illusion?* ed. A. Noë, 13–16. Thorverton, UK: Academic Imprint.

Descartes, R. [1637] 1902. *La Dioptrique*. In *Oeuvres de Descartes*, vol. 6, ed C. Adam and P. Tannery, 81–228. Paris: Cerf.

Descartes, R. [1637] 1965. *Discourse on Methods, Optics, Geometry and Meteorology*. Trans. P. J. Olscamp. New York: Bobbs-Merrill.

Descartes, R. [1641] 1988a. *Meditations on First Philosophy* in *The Principle Writings of Descartes, vol. II*, ed. John Cottingham, Robert Stoothoff, and Dugald Murdoch. Cambridge: Cambridge University Press, 1984.

Descartes, R. [1641] 1988b. *Objections and Replies* in *The Principle Writings of Descartes, vol. II*, ed. John Cottingham, Robert Stoothoff, and Dugald Murdoch. Cambridge: Cambridge University Press, 1984.

Ditchburn, R. W., and B. L. Ginsborg. 1952. Vision with a stabilized retinal image. *Nature* 170: 36–37.

Dretske, F. 1993. Conscious experience. *Mind* 102, no. 406: 263–283.

Dretske, F. 1995. *Naturalizing the Mind*. Cambridge, MA: The MIT Press.

Dretske, F. 2004. Change blindness. *Philosophical Studies* 120: 1–18.

Dreyfus, H. L. [1972] 1992. *What Computers Still Can't Do*. Cambridge, MA: The MIT Press.

Durgin, F. H., S. P. Tripathy, and D. M. Levi. 1995. On the filling in of the visual blind spot: Some rules of thumb. *Perception* 24, no. 7: 827–840.

Edelman, G. 1989. *The Remembered Present*. New York: Basic Books.

Euclid. 1945 The optics of Euclid. Trans. H. E. Burton. *Journal of the Optical Society of America* 35: 357–372.

Evans, G. 1982. *The Varieties of Reference*. Oxford: Oxford University Press.

Evans, G. 1985. Molyneux's question. In *Collected Papers*, 364–399. Oxford: Oxford University Press.

Fodor, J. A. 1975. *The Language of Thought*. Cambridge, MA: The MIT Press.

Fodor, J. A., and Z. W. Pylyshyn. 1981. How direct is visual perception? Some reflections on Gibson's "ecological approach." *Cognition* 9, 139–196. Reprinted in *Vision and Mind: Selected Readings in the Philosophy of Perception*, ed. A. Noë and E. Thompson, 167–227. Cambridge, MA: The MIT Press, 2002.

Frege, G. [1879] 1980. Begriffsschrift. In *Translations from the Philosophical Writings of Gotlob Frege*, 3rd ed., ed. P. Geach and M. Black. Oxford: Basil Blackwell.

Frege, G. [1884] 1950. *The Foundations of Arithmetic*. Trans. by J. L. Austin. Oxford: Basil Blackwell.

Frege, G. [1918–1919] 1984. Thoughts. In *Collected Papers on Mathematics, Logic and Philosophy*, ed. B. McGuinness, 351–372. Oxford: Basil Blackwell.

Gallagher, S. 2003. Bodily self-awareness and object-perception. *Theoria et Historia Scientiarum: International Journal for Interdisciplinary Studies* 7, no. 1: 53–68.

Gibson, J. J. 1979. *The Ecological Approach to Visual Perception*. Hillsdale, NJ: Lawrence Erlbaum.

Gibson, J. J., and D. Wadell. Homogeneous retina stimulation and visual perception. *American Journal of Psychology* 64: 263–270.

Gombrich, E. 1960–1961. *Art and Illusion: A Study in the Art of Pictorial Representation*. Princeton, NJ: Princeton University Press.

Gregory, R. L. [1966] 1997. *Eye and Brain: The Psychology of Seeing*, 5th ed. New York: McGraw-Hill.

Gregory, R. L., and J. G. Wallace. 1963. Recovery from early blindness: A case study. *Experimental Psychology Society*. Mongraph no. 2.

Grice, H. P. 1961. The causal theory of perception. *Proceedings of the Aristotelian Society*, suppl. vol. 35: 121–152.

Grice, H. P. 1962. Some remarks about the senses. In *Analytic Philosophy*, ed. R. J. Butler, 133–153. Oxford: Basil Blackwell. Reprinted in *Vision and Mind: Selected Readings in the Philosophy of Perception*, ed. A. Noë and E. Thompson, 35–54. Cambridge, MA: The MIT Press, 2002.

Grimes, J. 1996. On the failure to detect changes in scenes across saccades. In *Perception: Vancouver Studies in Cognitive Science*, vol. 2, ed. K. Akins, 89–110. Oxford: Oxford University Press.

Hacker, P. M. S. 1987. *Appearance and Reality*. Oxford: Basil Blackwell.

Hardin, C. L. 1986. *Color for Philosophers: Unweaving the Rainbow*. Indianapolis: Hackett.

Harman, G. 1990. The intrinsic quality of experience. In *Philosophical Perspectives 4*, ed. J. Tomberlin, 31–52. Northridge, CA: Ridgeview.

Harris, C. 1965. Perceptual adaptation to inverted, reversed, and displaced vision. *Psychological Review* 72, no. 6: 419–444.

Harris, C. 1980. "Insight or out of sight?: Two examples of perceptual plasticity in the human adult. In *Visual Coding and Adaptability*, ed. Charles S. Harris, 95–149. Hillsdale, NJ: Lawrence Erlbaum.

Hayes, A., and J. Ross. 1995. Lines of sight. In *The Artful Eye*, ed. R. Gregory, J. Harris, P. Heard, and D. Rose, 339–352. New York: Oxford University Press.

Heck, R. 2000. Non-conceptual content and the 'space of reasons.' *Philosophical Review* 109: 483–523.

Held, R., and A. Hein. 1963. Movement produced stimulation in the development of visually guided behavior. *Journal of Comparative and Physiological Psychology* 56: 873–876.

Hochberg, J. E., W. Triebel, and G. Seaman. 1951. Color adaptation under conditions of homogeneous visual stimulation (Ganzfeld). *Journal of Experimental Psychology* 41: 153–159.

Hume, D. [1739–1740] 1975. *A Treatise of Human Nature*, 2nd ed., ed. L. A. Selby-Bigge, rev. P. H. Nidditch. Oxford: Clarendon Press.

Humphrey, N. 1992. *A History of the Mind*. New York: Simon & Schuster.

Hurley, S. L. 1998. *Consciousness in Action*. Cambridge, MA: Harvard University Press.

Hurley, S. L. 2001. Overintellectualizing the mind. *Philosophy and Phenomenological Research* 63: 423–431.

Hurley, S. L., and A. Noë. 2003a. Neural plasticity and consciousness. *Biology and Philosophy* 18: 131–168.

Hurley, S. L., and A. Noë. 2003b. Neural plasticity and consciousness: Reply to Block. *Trends in Cognitive Sciences* 7, no. 8 (August): 342.

Hurvich, L. 1981. *Colour Vision*. Sunderland, MA: Sinauer.

Husserl, E. [1907] 1997. *Thing and Space: Lectures of 1907*. Trans. Richard Rojcewicz. Boston: Kluwer.

Hyman, J. 1989. *The Imitation of Nature*. Oxford: Basil Blackwell.

Ittelson, W. H. 1952. *The Ames Demonstrations in Perception*. Oxford: Oxford University Press.

Jackson, F. 1982. Epiphenomenal qualia. *Philosophical Quarterly* 32: 127–136.

Jackson, F. 1986. What Mary didn't know. *Journal of Philosophy* 83: 291–295.

Järvilehto, T. 1998a. The theory of the organism-environment system: I. Description of the theory. *Integrative Physiological and Behavioral Science* 33: 317–330.

Järvilehto, T. 1998b. The theory of the organism-environment system: II. Significance of nervous activity in the organism-environment system. *Integrative Physiological and Behavioral Science* 33: 331–338.

Järvilehto, T. 1999. The theory of the organism-environment system: III. Role of efferent influences on receptors in the formation of knowledge. *Integrative Physiological and Behavioral Science* 34: 90–100.

Järvilehto, T. 2000. The theory of the organism-environment system: IV. The problem of mental activity and consciousness. *Integrative Physiological and Behavioral Science* 35: 35–57.

Jeannerod, M. 1997. *The Cognitive Neuroscience of Action*. Oxford: Blackwell.

Johnston, M. 1992. How to speak of the colors. *Philosophical Studies* 68: 221–263.

Jonas, H. 1966. The nobility of sight: A study in the phenomenology of the senses. In *The Phenomenon of Life*. New York: Harper & Row.

Kant, I. [1781–1987] 1929. *Critique of Pure Reason*. Trans. Norman Kemp Smith. London: Macmillan.

Kauffman, S. 1995. *At Home in the Universe*. New York: Oxford University Press.

Kaufman, T., H. Théoret, and A. Pascual-Leone. 2002. Braille character discrimination in blindfolded human subjects. *Neuroreport* 13, no. 16: 1–4.

Keeley, B. 2001. Making sense of the senses. *Journal of Philosophy* 99, no. 1: 1–24.

Kelly, S. D. Forthcoming. Seeing things in Merleau-Ponty. In *Cambridge Companion to Merleau-Ponty*. Cambridge: Cambridge University Press.

Kelly, S. D. 2001. The non-conceptual content of perceptual experience: Situation dependence and fineness of grain. *Philosophy and Phenomenological Research* 62, no. 3: 601–608.

Kelso, S. J. A. 1995. *Dynamic Patterns: The Self-Organization of Brain and Behavior*. Cambridge, MA: The MIT Press.

Kenny, A. [1971] 1984. The homunculus fallacy. In *The Legacy of Wittgenstein*, 125–136. Oxford: Blackwell.

Kenny, A. 1989. *The Metaphysics of Mind*. Oxford: Oxford University Press.

Kepler, J. 1964. De modo visionis. Trans. A. C. Crombie. In *Mélange Alexandre Koyré,* vol. 1, *L'aventure de la science,* 135–172. Paris: Hermann.

Koch, C. 2004. *The Quest for Consciousness: A Neurobiological Approach*. Englewood, CO: Roberts & Co.

Koenderink, J. J. 1984a. The concept of local sign. In *Limits in Perception,* ed. A. J. van Doorn, W. A. van de Grind, and J. J. Koenderink, 495–547. Zeist, Netherlands: VNU Science Press.

Koenderink, J. J. 1984b. The internal representation of solid shape and visual exploration. In *Sensory experience, adaptation, and perception. Festschrift for Ivo Kohler,* ed. L. Spillmann and B. R. Wooten, 123–142. Hillsdale, NJ: Lawrence Erlbaum.

Kohler, I. [1951] 1964. Formation and transformation of the perceptual world. *Psychological Issues* 3, no. 4: 1–173.

Krauskopf, J. 1963. Effects of retinal stabilization on the appearance of heterochromatic targets. *Journal of the Optical Society of America* 53: 741–744.

Langer, M. S., and A. Gilchrist. 2000. Color perception in a 3-D scene of one reflectance. *Investigative Ophthalmology & Visual Science* 41: 1254B629.

Lettvin, J. Y., H. R. Maturana, W. S. McCulloch, and W. H. Pitts. 1959. What the frog's eye tells the frog's brain. *Proceedings of the Institute of Radio Engineers.* 47: 1940–1951. Reprinted in *Embodiments of Mind,* ed. Warren S. McCulloch. Cambridge, MA: The MIT Press, 1965.

Levin, D. T. 2002. Change blindness blindness as visual metacognition. *Journal of Consciousness Studies* 9: 5–6: 111–130.

Levin, D. T., N. Momen, S. B. Drwdahl, and D. J. Simons. 2000. Change blindness blindness: The meta-cognitive error of overestimating change-detection ability. *Visual Cognition* 7 (1.2.3): 397–412.

Levin, D. T., D. J. Simons, B. L. Angelone, and C. F. Chabris. 2002. Memory for centrally attended changing objects in an incidental real-world change detection paradigm. *British Journal of Psychology* 93: 289–302.

Lewis, D. 1980. Veridical hallucination and prosthetic vision. *Australasian Journal of Philosophy* 58: 239–249. Reprinted in *Vision and Mind: Selected Readings in the Philosophy of Perception,* ed. A. Noë and E. Thompson, 135–150. Cambridge, MA: The MIT Press, 2002.

Lindberg, D. C. 1976. *Theories of Vision from Al-Kindi to Kepler*. Chicago: University of Chicago Press.

Locke, J. [1689] 1975. *An Essay Concerning Human Understanding.* Ed. and with an introduction by Peter H. Nidditch. Oxford: Oxford University Press.

Mach, E. [1886] 1959. *The Analysis of Sensation.* Trans. C. M. Williams. New York: Dover.

Mack, A., and I. Rock. 1998. *Inattentional Blindness.* Cambridge, MA: The MIT Press.

MacKay, D. M. 1962. Theoretical models of space perception. In *Aspects of the Theory of Artificial Intelligence,* ed. C. A. Muses, 83–104. New York: Plenum.

MacKay, D. M. 1967. Ways of looking at perception. In *Models for the Perception of Speech and Visual Form,* ed. W. Wathen-Dunn, 25–43. Cambridge, MA: The MIT Press.

MacKay, D. M. 1973. Visual stability and voluntary eye movements. In *Handbook of sensory physiology,* vol. VII/3A, ed. R. Jung, 307–331. Berlin: Springer.

Marr, D. 1982. *Vision.* New York: W. H. Freeman and Sons.

Martin, M. 1992. Sight and touch. In *The Contents of Experience: Essays on Perception,* ed. T. Crane, 196–215. Cambridge: Cambridge University Press.

Martin, M. 2002. The transparency of experience. In *Mind and Language* 17: 376–425.

Maturana, H. R., and F. J. Varela. 1987. *The Tree of Knowledge: The Biological Roots of Human Understanding,* rev. ed. Boston: Shambhala.

McClintock, M. K. 1971. Menstrual synchrony and suppression. *Nature* 229: 244–245.

McDowell, J. 1982. Criteria, defeasibility and knowledge. *Proceedings of the British Academy* 68: 455–79.

McDowell, J. 1986. Singular thought and the extent of inner space. In *Subject, Thought and Context,* ed. P. Pettit and J. McDowell, 137–168. Oxford: Oxford University Press.

McDowell, J. 1994a. *Mind and World.* Cambridge, MA: Harvard University Press.

McDowell, J. 1994b. The content of perceptual experience. *Philosophical Quarterly* 44, no. 175: 190–205. Reprinted in *Vision and Mind: Selected Readings in the Philosophy of Perception,* ed. A. Noë and E. Thompson, 443–458. Cambridge, MA: The MIT Press, 2002.

Meijer, P. B. L . 1992. An experimental system for auditory image representations. *IEEE Transactions on Biomedical Engineering* 39, no. 2: 112–121. Reprinted in the *1993 IMIA Yearbook of Medical Informatics,* ed. J. Bemmel and A. T. McCray, 291–300. Stuttgart: Schattauer Publishing House, Inc.

Merleau-Ponty, M. [1945] 1962. *The Phenomenology of Perception*. Trans. Colin Smith. London: Routledge Press, 1962.

Merleau-Ponty, M. 1964. *L'Oeil et L'Esprit*. Paris: Gallimard.

Merleau-Ponty, M. [1948] 1973. *The Visible and the Invisible*. Trans. Alphonso Lingis. Evanston, IL: Northwestern University Press.

Merzenich, M. 2000. Seeing in the sound zone. *Nature* 404: 820–821.

Metzger, W. 1930 Optische Untersuchungen in Ganzfeld II. *Psychlogische Forschung* 13: 6–29.

Milner, A. D., and M. A. Goodale. 1998. Precis of *Visual Brain in Action*. *Psyche* 4, no. 12: 515–529. Available at http://psyche.cs.monash.edu.au/v4/psyche-4-12-milner.html. Reprinted in *Vision and Mind: Selected Readings in the Philosophy of Perception*, ed. A. Noë and E. Thompson, 515–529. Cambridge, MA: The MIT Press, 2002.

Minsky, M. 1985. *The Society of Mind*. New York: Simon & Schuster.

Mitroff, S. R., D. J. Simons, and D. T. Levin. Forthcoming. Nothing compares 2 views: Change blindness can occur despite preserved access to the changed information. *Perception and Psychophysics*.

Murakami, I., and P. Cavanagh. 2001. Visual jitter: Evidence for visual-motion-based compensation of retinal slip due to small eye movements. *Visual Research* 41: 173–186.

Murakami, I. 1995. Motion aftereffect after monocular adaptation to filled-in motion at the blind spot. *Vision Research* 35: 1041–1045.

Nakayama, K. 1994. Gibson: an appreciation. *Psychological Review* 101, no. 2: 353–356.

Neisser, U. 1976. *Cognition and reality: Principles and implications of cognitive psychology*. San Francisco: W. H. Freeman.

Newton, I. [1704] 1952. *Opticks*, 4th ed. New York: Dover.

Noë, A. 1995. *Experience and the Mind: An Essay on the Metaphysics of Experience*. Cambridge, MA: Harvard University, UMI Dissertation Services.

Noë, A. 2001. Experience and the active mind. *Synthese* 29: 41–60.

Noë, A. 2001b. Experience and experiment in art. *Journal of Consciousness Studies* 7, nos. 8–9: 123–135.

Noë, A. 2002a. On what we see. *Pacific Philosophical Quarterly* 83: 1.

Noë, A. 2002b. Is perspectival self-consciousness nonconceptual? *The Philosophical Quarterly* 52, no. 207 (April): 185–194.

Noë, A. 2002c. Is the visual world a grand illusion? *Is the Visual World a Grand Illusion?*, ed. A. Noë, 1–12. Thorverton, UK: Imprint Academic.

Noë, A. 2002d. Direct perception. *The Macmillan Encyclopedia of Cognitive Science.* London: Macmillan.

Noë, A. 2003. Perception and causation: the puzzle unraveled. *Analysis* 63, no. 2 (April): 93–100.

Noë, A. 2005. Experience without the head. In *Perceptual Experience,* ed. T. S. Gendler and J. Hawthorne. Oxford: Oxford University Press.

Noë, A., and S. L. Hurley. 2003. The deferential brain in action. Reply to Jeffrey Gray. *Trends in Cognition Sciences* 7, no. 5 (May): 195–196.

Noë, A., and J. K. O'Regan. 2000. Perception, attention and the grand illusion. *Psyche* 6, no. 15. Available at http://psyche.cs.monash.edu.au/v6/psyche-6-15-noe.html.

Noë, A., and J. K. O'Regan. 2002. On the brain basis of perceptual consciousness. In A. *Vision and Mind: Selected Readings in the Philosophy of Perception,* ed. A. Noë and E. Thompson, 567–598. Cambridge, MA: The MIT Press.

Noë, A., and E. Thompson. 2004a. Are there neural correlates of consciousness? *Journal of Consciousness Studies* 11, no.1: 3–28.

Noë, A., and E. Thompson. 2004b. Sorting out the neural basis of consciousness. *Journal of Consciousness Studies* 11, no. 1: 87–98.

Noë, A., L. Pessoa, and E. Thompson. 2000. Beyond the grand illusion: What change blindness really teaches us about vision. *Visual Cognition* 7: 93–106.

Noë, A., and E. Thompson. 2002. *Vision and Mind: Selected Readings in the Philosophy of Perception.* Cambridge, MA: The MIT Press.

O'Callaghan, C. 2002. *Sounds as Events.* Ph.D. diss., Princeton University.

O'Regan, J. K. 1992. Solving the "real" mysteries of visual perception: The world as an outside memory. *Canadian Journal of Psychology* 46, no. 3: 461–488.

O'Regan, J. K., and A. Noë. 2001c. What it is like to see: A sensorimotor theory of perceptual experience. *Synthese:* 29: 79–103.

O'Regan, J. K., and A. Noë. 2001a. A sensorimotor approach to vision and visual consciousness. *Behavioral and Brain Sciences* 24, no. 5: 939–973.

O'Regan, J. K., and A. Noë. 2001b. Authors' response: Acting out our sensory experience. *Behavioral and Brain Sciences* 24, 5: 1011–1030.

O'Regan, J. K., H. Deubel, J. J. Clark, and R. A. Rensink. 2000. Picture changes during blinks: Looking without seeing and seeing without looking. *Visual Cognition* 7 (1.2.3): 191–212.

O'Regan, J. K., E. Myin, and A. Noë. Forthcoming. Toward an analytic phenomenology: The concept of "bodiliness" and "grabbiness." *Seeing and Thinking: Reflections on Kanizsa's Studies in Visual Cognition,* ed. A. Carsetti. London: Kluwer.

O'Regan, J. K., J. A. Rensink, and J. J. Clark. 1996. "Mud splashes" render picture changes invisible. *Investigative Ophthalmology and Visual Science* 37: S213.

O'Regan, J. K., R. A. Rensink, and J. J. Clark. 1999. Change-blindness as a result of 'mudsplashes'. *Nature* 398: 34.

O'Shaughnessy, B. 1980. *The Will,* vols. 1 and 2. Cambridge: Cambridge University Press.

O'Shaughnessy, B. 2000. *Consciousness and the World.* New York: Oxford University Press.

Pallas, S. L., and M. Sur. 1993. Visual projections induced into the auditory pathway of ferrets: II. Coriticocoritical connections of primary auditory cortex. *Journal of Comparative Neurology* 337, no. 2: 317–333.

Palmer, S. 1999a. *Vision: From Photons to Phenomenology.* Cambridge, MA: The MIT Press.

Palmer, S. 1999b. Color, consciousness, and the isomorphism constraint. *Behavioral & Brain Sciences* 22, no. 6: 923–943.

Paradiso, M. A., and K. Nakayama. 1991. Brightness perception and filling-in. *Vision Research* 31: 1221–1236.

Pascual-Leone, A., and R. Hamilton. The metamodal organization of the brain. In *Vision: From Neurons to Cognition* (Progress in Brain Research, vol. 134.), ed. C. Casanova and M. Ptito, 427–445. Amsterdam: Elsevier Science.

Peacocke, C. 1983. *Sense and Content.* Oxford: Oxford University Press.

Peacocke, C. 1987. Depiction. *Philosophical Review* 96: 383–410.

Peacocke, C. 1992. *Concepts.* Cambridge, MA: The MIT Press.

Peacocke, C. 2001. Does Perception have a nonconceptual content? *Journal of Philosophy* 98: 239–264.

Penfield, W., and Jasper, H. 1954. *Epilepsy and the functional anatomy of the human brain.* Boston: Little, Brown.

Pessoa, L., E. Thompson, and A. Noe. 1998. Finding out about filling: A guide to perceptual completion for visual science and the philosophy of perception. *Behavioral & Brain Sciences* 21, no. 6: 723–802.

Pettit, P. 2003a. Looks red. *Philosophical Issues* 13, no. 1: 221–252.

Pettit, P. 2003b. Motion blindness and the knowledge argument. In *The Knowledge Argument,* ed. P. Ludlow, Y. Nagasawa, and D. Stoljar. Cambridge, MA: The MIT Press.

Pinker, S. 1997. *How the Mind Works.* New York: W. W. Norton.

Plato. 1929. *Timaeus. Critias. Cleitophon. Menexus. Eipisteles*. Trans. R. G. Bury. (Loeb Classical Library, Plato, vol. IX.) Cambridge, MA: Harvard University Press.

Poincaré, H. [1902] 1952. *Science and Hypothesis*. Preface by J. Larmor. New York: Dover.

Poincaré, H. [1905] 1958. *The Value of Science*. Trans. G. B. Halstead. New York: Dover.

Price, H. H. 1948. *Hume's Theory of the External World*. Oxford: Clarendon Press.

Priest, S. 1998. *Merleau-Ponty*. London: Routledge.

Ptolemy, C. 1956. *L'Optique de Claude Ptolémée dans las version latine d'apres l'arabe de l'émir eugene de Sicile*, ed. Albert Lejeune. Louvain: Université de Louvain.

Putnam, H. 1963. Brains and behavior. In *Analytic Philosophy*, 2nd series, ed. R. J. Butler, 1–19. Oxford: Basil Blackwell and Mott.

Putnam, H. 1992. *Renewing Philosophy*. Cambridge, MA: Harvard University Press.

Putnam, H. 1999. *The Threefold Cord: Mind, Body, World*. New York: Columbia University Press.

Pylyshyn, Z. W. 2001. Seeing, acting, and knowing. [Commentary on O'Regan and Noë 2001.] *Behavioral and Brain Sciences* 24, no. 5: 999.

Ramachandran, V. S., and S. Blakeslee. 1998. *Phantoms in the Brain*. New York: William Morrow & Co.

Rensink, R. 2000. The dynamic representation of scenes. *Visual Cognition* 7 (1.2.3): 17–42.

Rensink, R. A., J. K. O'Regan, and J. J. Clark. 1997. To see or not to see: The need for attention to perceive changes in scenes. *Psychological Science* 8, no. 5: 368–373.

Rensink, R. A., J. K. O'Regan, and J. J. Clark. 2000. On the failure to detect changes in scenes across brief interruptions. *Visual Cognition* 7, no. 1: 127–146.

Riggs, L. A., F. Ratliff, J. C. Cornsweet, and T. N. Cornsweet. 1953. The disappearance of steadily fixated visual test objects. *Journal of the Optical Society of America* 43: 495–501.

Roe, A. W., S. L. Pallas, J-O. Hahm, and M. Sur. 1990. A map of visual space induced in primary auditory cortex. *Science* 250, no. 4982: 818–820.

Roe, Anna W., S. L. Pallas, Y. H. Kwon, and M. Sur. 1992. Visual projections routed to the auditory pathway in ferrets. *Journal of Neuroscience* 12, no. 9: 3651–3664.

Rossetti, Y., C. Pisella, and A. Vighetta. 2003. Optic ataxia revisited: Visual guided action versus immediate visuomotor control. *Experimental and Brain Research* 153: 171–179.

Rowlands, M. 2002. The dogmas of consciousness. In *Is the Visual World a Grand Illusion?*, 158–180. Thorverton, UK: Imprint Academic.

Rowlands, M. 2003. *Externalism: Putting Mind and World Together Again*. Chesham, UK: Acumen.

Ruskin, J. [1856] 1971. *The Elements of Drawing*. New York: Dover.

Ryle, G. [1949] 1990. *The Concept of Mind*. London: Penguin Books.

Sabra, A. I. 1989. *The Optics of Iba al-Haytham: Books I–III: On Direct Vision*. Trans. with an introduction and commentary by A. I. Sabra. London: Warburg Institute.

Sacks, O. 1995. *An Anthropologist on Mars: Seven Paradoxical Tales*. New York: Knopf.

Sadato, N., A. Pascual-Leone, J. Grafman, M. P. Deiber, V. Ibanez, and M. Hallett. 1998. Neural networks for Braille reading by the blind. *Brain* 121, no. 7: 1213–1229.

Sadato, N., A. Pascual-Leone, J. Grafman, J., V. Ibanez, M. P. Deiber, G. Dold, and M. Hallett. 1996. Activation of the primary visual cortex by Braille reading in blind subjects. *Nature* 380, no. 6574: 526–528.

Sanford, D. 1997. Some puzzles about prosthetic perception. Paper presented at the 1997 meetings of the Society for Philosophy and Psychology, New York.

Scheiner, C. 1919. *Oculus, hoc est fundamentum opticum* . . . Innsbruck: Agricola.

Schone, H. 1962. Optische gesteuerte Lageänderungen (Versuche an Dytiscidenlarren zur Vertikelorientierong.) *Z. Verg. Physiol.* 45: 590–604.

Searle, J. 1983. *Intentionality: An Essay in the Philosophy of Mind*. Cambridge: Cambridge University Press.

Searle, J. 1992. *The Rediscovery of Mind*. Cambridge, MA: The MIT Press.

Searle. J. 2000. *Annual Review of Neuroscience* 23: 557–578.

Searle, J. 2004. Comments on "Are there neural correlates of consciousness?" *Journal of Consciousness Studies* 11, no. 1: 80–82.

Sellars, W. 1956. Empiricism and the philosophy of mind. In *Minnesota Studies in the Philosophy of Science*, vol. 2, ed. H. Feigl and M. Scriven, 253–329. Minneapolis: University of Minnesota Press.

Shapiro, L. A. 2000. Multiple realization. *Journal of Philosophy* 97, no. 12: 635–654.

Sharma, J., A. Angelucci, and M. Sur. 2000. Induction of visual orientation modules in auditory cortex. *Nature* 404, no. 6780: 841–847.

Shimojo, S., Y. Kamitani, and S. Nishida. 2001. Afterimage of perceptually filled-in surfaces. *Science* 293: 1677–1680.

Shoemaker, S. 1968. Self-reference and self-awareness. *Journal of Philosophy* 65: 555–567.

Shoemaker, S. 1982. The inverted spectrum. *Journal of Philosophy* 79: 357–381.

Siewert, C. 2004. Is experience transparent? *Philosophical Studies* 117: 15–41.

Simons, D. J., and C. F. Chabris. 1999. Gorillas in our midst: Sustained inattentional blindness for dynamic events. *Perception* 28: 1059–1074.

Simons, D. J., and D. T. Levin. 1997. Change blindness. *Trends in Cognitive Sciences* 1, no. 7: 261–267.

Simons, D. J., and D. T. Levin. 1998. Failure to detect change during real-world interaction. *Psychonomic Bulletin and Review* 5: 644–649.

Simons, D. J., C. F Chabris, T. T. Schnur, and D. T. Levin. 2002. Evidence for preserved representations in change blindness. *Consciousness and Cognition* 11: 78–97.

Snowdon, P. 1980–1981. Perception, vision and causation. *Proceedings of the Aristotelian Society* 81: 175–192. Reprinted in *Vision and Mind: Selected Readings in the Philosophy of Perception,* ed. A. Noë and E. Thompson, 151–166. Cambridge, MA: The MIT Press.

Stanley, S., and T. Williamson. 2001. Knowing how. *Journal of Philosophy* 98: 411–444.

Stoljar, D. Forthcoming. The argument from diaphonousness. In *New Essays in the Philosophy of Language and Mind,* suppl. to *The Canadian Journal of Philosophy,* ed. M. Ezcurdia, R. Stainton, and C. Viger. Calgary: University of Calgary Press.

Stratton, G. M. 1897. Vision without inversion of the retinal image. *Psychological Review* 4: 341–360, 463–481.

Strawson, G. 1989. Red and 'red'. *Synthese* 78: 193–232.

Strawson, P. F. 1959. *Individuals.* London: Methuen.

Strawson, P. F. 1974. Causation in perception. In *Freedom and Resentment and Other Essays.* London: Methuen.

Strawson, P. F. 1979. Perception and its objects. In *Perception and Identity: Essays Presented to A. J. Ayer with His Replies,* ed. G. F. MacDonald, 41–60. Ithaca: Cornell University Press. Reprinted in *Vision and Mind: Selected Readings in the Philosophy of Perception,* ed. A. Noë and E. Thompson, Cambridge, 91–110. Cambridge, MA: The MIT Press, 2002.

Sur, M., A. Angelucci, and J. Sharma. 1999. Rewiring cortex: The role of patterned activity in development and plasticity of neocortical circuits. *Journal of Neurobiology* 41, no. 1: 33–43.

Taylor, J. G. 1962. *The Behavioral Basis of Perception.* New Haven, CT: Yale University Press.

Thompson, E. 1995. *Colour Vision.* London: Routledge.

Thompson, E. Forthcoming. *Radical Embodiment: The Lived Body in Biology, Human Experience, and the Sciences of the Mind.* Cambridge, MA: Harvard University Press.

Thompson, E., and F. J. Varela 2001. Radical embodiment: Neural dynamics and consciousness. *Trends in Cognitive Sciences* 5: 418–425.

Thompson, E., A. Noe, and L. Pessoa. 1999. Perceptual completion: A case study in phenomenology and cognitive science. In *Naturalizing Phenomenology: Issues in Contemporary Phenomenology and Cognitive Science,* ed. J. Petitot, J-M. Roy, B. Pachoud, and F. J. Varela. Palo Alto, CA: Stanford University Press.

Thompson, E., A. Palacios, and F. Varela. 1992. Ways of coloring: Comparative color vision as a case study for cognitive science. *Behavioral and Brain Sciences* 19: 1–74. Reprinted in *Vision and Mind,* ed. A. Noe and E. Thompson, 351–418. Cambridge, MA: The MIT Press, 2002.

Toombs, S. K. 1992. *The Meaning of Illness: A Phenomenological Account of the Different Perspectives on Physician and Patient.* Dordrecht: Kluwer.

Tye, M. 2000. *Consciousness, Color, and Content.* Cambridge, MA: The MIT Press.

Ullman, S. 1980. Against direct perception. *Behavioral & Brain Sciences* 3: 373–415.

Valvo, A. 1971. *Sight Restoration after Long-Term Blindness: the Problems and Behavior Patterns of Visual Rehabilitation.* New York: American Federation for the Blind.

Varela, F. J., E. Thompson, and E. Rosch. 1991. *The Embodied Mind.* Cambridge, MA: The MIT Press.

von Senden, M. [1932] 1960. *Space and Sight.* Trans. Peter Heath. London: Methuen.

Wade, N. J. 1998. *A Natural History of Vision.* Cambridge, MA: The MIT Press.

Weiskrantz, L. 1978. *Blindsight.* Oxford: Oxford University Press.

Westphal, J. 1987. *Colour: A Philosophical Introduction.* Oxford: Basil Blackwell.

Wittgenstein, L. [1930] 1975. *Philosophical Remarks,* ed. R. Rhees. Trans. R. Hargreaves and R. White. Oxford: Blackwell.

Wittgenstein, L. 1953 *Philosophical Investigations,* 3rd ed. Trans. G. E. M. Anscombe. Oxford: Blackwell.

Wittgenstein, L. 1958. *The Blue and the Brown Books.* Oxford: Blackwell.

Wollheim, R. [1968] 1980. *Art and Its Objects,* 2nd ed. Cambridge: Cambridge University Press.

Wollheim, R. 1998. On pictorial representation. *Journal of Aesthetics and Art Criticism* 56: 217–226.

Yarbus, A. L. 1967. *Eye Movements and Vision.* New York: Plenum.

Index